MW00624439

TITANS OF
DENTISTRY

TITANS OF DENTISTRY

How the Top Performers Think and Act Differently

by Justin Short and David Maloley

Copyright © 2018 by Dr Justin Short & Dr David Maloley

All rights reserved. No part of this publication
may be reproduced or transmitted by any means,
without prior permission of the publisher.

ISBN: 978-0-9997863-3-8

Published by Soapbox Books

Dedicated To

Bennett Maloley &
Reese, Rowan, and Truman Short.

Your dads are excited to see the
Titans you become!

CONTENTS

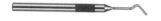

PROLOGUE

*"He who walks with the wise will be wise,
but a companion of fools will suffer harm."*

—PROVERBS—

I was sitting on the deck of our rental house on Longboat Key, FL in the winter of 2017. A ten-day escape with my wife and kids from the harsh reality of winter in St. Louis where we live. As I was enjoying the sunshine, I was putting the finishing touches on a weekly email I send out to everyone on my email list for The Lifestyle Practice—a dental coaching company I began the year prior.

This particular email was an interview of someone who I viewed as a top performer in our profession of dentistry. I say "our" because if you're not a dentist or in the dental field, you must be extremely hard up for material to pick up a book called *Titans of Dentistry*. As I hit send, as I do almost every week, my phone went off on the table next to me. A text message. It was Dr. Dave Maloley. The original *Relentless Dentist.*

Dave and I were becoming fast friends. He had followed my weekly broadcast for awhile, I had followed and been on his podcast, and Dave was even one of the docs I interviewed for the series I was doing featuring top performers.

He mentioned how he was really enjoying this collection, which covered how top performers thought and acted differently on topics and situations all of us encounter. He then asked, "Have you ever considered writing a book like this?"

I replied, "You mean Titans of Dentistry? ☺", and from that day on, we've been slowly but steadily working on the project you're holding right now. We hope you enjoy it and that it pushes and inspires you to do great things outside of, and within, our wonderful profession.

– Dr. Justin Short, The Lifestyle Practice

INTRODUCTION

Merriam-Webster defines Titan as "one that stands out for greatness of achievement". In fact, that is exactly who and what we looked for to include in this book. The doctors or *Titans*, as we've lovingly dubbed them, included in this book are by no means the only ones out there. We know there are many, many wonderful dentists. Some under the radar, and some not. In fact, there were many dentists not featured in the book that could have been or should have been—or that we would have liked to include, but due to time and space constraints, we had to narrow it down. Perhaps someday there will be a *Titans of Dentistry, Part Deux*.

Many of the *Titans* featured are people you will recognize, but some you may not. However, recognizable or not, we felt that they all stood out in one way or another for greatness of achievement.

Some are expert clinicians, many are educators or lecturers, some are dental podcasters, and some have incredibly successful single-location private practices. These doctors have practices all across North America. Some still practice hands-on dentistry, and some do not. Some run multi-million-dollar companies, and some a single location. They are all uncommon.

Our objective for this book was to dig deep to learn how these top performers and/or personalities think and act differently than the masses.

What is it that sets them apart?

How do they approach life and practice differently?

How do they handle setbacks that we all encounter?

What are their habits and routines?

How do they define success?

The list goes on, but in summation, are there commonalities they share that we can take away and learn from, or not? Ultimately are there thoughts, ideas, patterns, etc...that we can take and apply in our own practice and life?

We found the answer to both of these questions to be...Yes!

Who is this book for?

If I'm being completely honest, if no one else purchased or read this book, I'd still be content having put in the work to complete it. (Have you ever tried to track down 30+ busy, successful dentists for a 45-minute interview?? #noteasy!)

I've always been intrigued by the traits, habits, and mindsets of successful outliers. So for me personally, being able to pick the brain, so to speak, of these doctors was an amazing opportunity!

I was just an average student at best in dental school. I'd often prefer to skip class and work on learning how to run a successful business, as opposed to learning the chemical composition of amalgam. I'm not condoning those actions, but it is what it is.

After 12 years of private practice, I was able to sell my practice and retire from hands-on dentistry. Most people, when they hear that, assume I must have hated doing dentistry. That wasn't the case at all. It wasn't a dislike of running a practice that pushed me away; it was simply the pull of things I liked to do more.

I enjoy spending time with my wife and 3 children more. I enjoy working on outside investments more. I enjoy working with doctors to grow their practice and create the freedom I've been fortunate to have...more. I know, to some, retiring from hands-on is dental blasphemy. I'd say to each their own.

This book is for those like Dr. Dave and I who have the same interests. I'm going to take the liberty to assume that if you're reading this book, you either are, or have aspirations of, being uncommonly successful like those featured in the subsequent pages.

Our hope is that you are richly rewarded. Dave and I hope that you finish this book inspired and armed with tools and ideas to take back and grow your practice and life.

What I learned...

What is often the case with these types of projects is that you go into it expecting to find one thing and end up walking away with something completely different. This book was no exception.

Looking back now, I think in my mind I was expecting to find traits and habits with these doctors that were in a way almost superhuman. Even though deep down I knew better, I still think I expected to see growth patterns all pointing up and to the right. Watching the careers of many of these outliers, as I have over the past many years, it's understandable for one to assume it was easier for them in some way.

As an onlooker admiring from afar, it almost makes one feel better to assume these doctors had fewer obstacles than others would have had. It protects the pride to figure they just had a leg up. Maybe they just happened to be in the right place at the right time, and unlike countless others, success (however one defines it) just came more naturally for them.

Less me go ahead and burst those bubbles right now. As you will see in this book, almost all of those assumptions turned out to be completely false.

I look at success as an iceberg. We only see the top 10%. We often aren't privy to what's going on below the surface. When we see a speaker on stage, sold out seminars, someone on the cover of top dental publications, dentists enjoying more freedom and financial resources than others down the street—we're only seeing the top 10%.

What we don't see is the other 90%, which is often filled with hard work, late nights, early mornings, the trading of 'me' time to work on their craft, passing on social gatherings, the denial of defeat when the odds are stacked against them, and the many other unmentioned sacrifices. Those are the decisions that create distance from the rest of the pack.

In all the interviews, not one Titan had a story that went like this: "I achieved success overnight, and I did it by following the herd, making easy decisions, binge-watching Netflix, and giving up when I hit obstacles. In fact, it was easy!"

Au contraire! If that was their story, there would be no need for this book because everyone could and would be a Titan at that point.

I think we have a subconscious bias to *want* to believe there is something magical about those that achieve uncommon levels of success or notoriety.

Nietzsche said, "For if we think of genius as something magical, we are not obliged to compare ourselves and find ourselves lacking...To call someone 'divine' means: 'there is no need to compete.'"

In the book *Grit*, Angela Duckworth discusses how mythologizing natural talent lets us all off the hook, allowing us to relax into the status quo.

Our goal in this book is keep you from relaxing into the status quo and to spur you on to greatness, however you define it.

What we discovered during these interviews is that these dentists are not superhuman. Even those I assumed walked on water had their own setbacks. It turns out that the doctors in this book are as flawed and imperfect as you and I, and their path to success was rarely a straight line.

Ever since I began studying top performers, I have been led back to a common theme, time and time again, and this book was no different; and that commonality is: *Mindset trumps*.

What the doctors in this book do have in common is a shared optimism. They were not complacent in their approach, nor did they sit back and let things happen by chance. They have taken, made, and acted on the opportunities they were given along their journey. They have been able to identify their unique talents and gifts and build their success around them. They didn't give up.

As a very wise man (Billy Ocean, Circa 1986) once said, "When the going gets tough, the tough get going"...and that's exactly what they have done.

How this book is set-up...

This book is organized as a series of interviews. For the most part, with a few exceptions, you will see the questions we asked are universal to the group of Titans.

We've included some of our own thoughts or notes in some of the interviews to provide some backstory, emphasis, or insight into why we chose to interview this particular doctor, or some other side facts we thought you might find interesting.

Dr. Maloley has written the conclusion to the chapters. And in the Appendix, there is a list of the books mentioned in this book.

Originally Dave and I had planned *not* to include our interviews in the book. Right before we sent to the publisher, we decided we didn't want to miss out on the fun...so we changed our minds. Mine will follow my introduction here, and Dave's will come right before his conclusion at the end of book.

Some themes throughout the book will be obvious; some are more subtle. One of the most prominent themes that stood out to me was that of persistence and determination. As I was organizing the interviews I often found myself thinking...had this person not been a dentist, they still would have been uncommonly successful. Dentistry just happened to be the medium they chose.

As I conclude this intro and we begin this journey into the minds of these doctors, I want to leave you with a quote. I have read this quote weekly for almost half my life at this point, but thought it illustrated the feeling I was left with after reading these interviews myself, perfectly.

Nothing in the world can take the place of Persistence.
Talent will not; nothing is more
common than unsuccessful men with talent.
Genius will not; unrewarded genius is almost a proverb.
Education will not; the world
is full of educated derelicts. Persistence and
determination alone are omnipotent.

—CALVIN COOLIDGE

We hope this book encourages you to stay persistent and determined on your path towards greatness of achievement.

Enjoy!

—DR. JUSTIN SHORT, THE LIFESTYLE PRACTICE

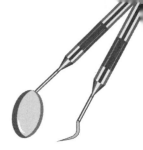

DR. JUSTIN SHORT

The Lifestyle Practice

Background

I'm originally from and still live in St. Louis, MO. What can I say, I'm a lifer. Although now at least we can spend our winters somewhere warm!

I graduated from St. Louis University and went on to dental school, graduating in 2005. I purchased a practice fairly soon after graduation, realizing I wasn't associate material. I owned 2 practices in my career. The time where I owned both simultaneously only overlapped for about a year. I grew the first one, and sold it. Grew the second...and sold it. My goal going into my career was to be "retired" by age 40. I sold my practice and retired from hands-on dentistry in 2017, at age 38. Not because I hated dentistry, but because I enjoyed the freedom of not having to go to an office anymore, and I had gotten to a point where I didn't HAVE to do it any longer for financial security.

Since I'm sure I will do some type of work until I die, because I enjoy what I do, I've always considered "retirement" to be when you don't have to be at a certain place for a certain amount of time each day to make your money.

Now I get to spend a good portion of my time with my wife and 3 children, who I adore. My kids are homeschooled, which now allows us a lot of freedom to travel and just be together. In 2016, I started a dental coaching company, The Lifestyle Practice. It keeps me busy, but I love working with docs to grow their practice, and to set and accomplish their personal vision for their lives. So to me, it isn't work.

I also invest in real estate a fair amount. I used the capital my practices provided as the fuel to grow our rental portfolio, which was/is a big reason I was able to sell and walk away from hands-on. Again, I enjoy it so much it never seems like work.

Please explain your style of practice (practice size, location, procedure mix, etc.)

We've all heard the term work/life balance in which our life gets the leftovers once our work is completed. While building my practices, I always tried to reverse that. I focused first on building the life I wanted, and then worked to design my practices around that.

My practices were both bread-and-butter practices. I did the occasional slam-dunk implant, clear aligner, and smile cases, but overall we focused on nailing the simple things we as dentists do day after day.

I attribute the success I had as a practice owner more to leadership and relationship building than breadth of procedures mix. For the last 10 years of my 12-year career, I worked 3 days a week, and when I sold my practice, I was taking at least 10 weeks off a year while gross production was close to $2M with 5 team members. That was my vision.

Do you have a favorite success quote or mantra?

If I had to pick a life mantra, it would have to be the verse I have a tattoo of. (Knock it off, we were all 18 once!) For the record, it's only the reference—"Joshua 1:9"—not the entire verse written out. Joshua 1:9 says, "Have I not commanded you? Be strong and courageous. Do not be afraid; do not be discouraged, for the Lord your God will be with you wherever you go."

Finally my dad constantly engrained in me, "You have to make hay, while you can make hay." I cannot count the number of times that ran through my head either at the end of a busy day when an EM patient comes in and needs a RCT/crown and I just wanted to go home, or you open up the distal of #19 and see a lesion on the mesial of 18 and just want to tell a patient, "We'll get that next time."

Hay also does not refer only to money. Perhaps you have the chance to brighten someone's day, or take your kids to lunch…take advantage of the opportunities as you have them. You never know what tomorrow will bring, so always try to make "hay" when you can.

In regards to your dental career, what would you like your legacy to be, or how would you like to be remembered?

Without a doubt, I'd like to be remembered for helping other doctors achieve the practices and lives they've always wanted, and to be able to enjoy the freedom that goes along with those things!

What does success mean to you?

I know we all have different definitions of success. I tend to divide it into categories. For example…personal and professional.

Personally, I want to have a healthy marriage, and children that know how much their dad loves them, and that love Jesus.

Professionally for me, it was to have financial freedom at a young age so that I could do what I want, with who I want, when I want.

If I would have had to choose between the two, I would have chosen the former, not the latter.

What is your morning routine (first 1–2 hrs of the day)?

Coffee. That's a constant. Other than that, my days vary quite a bit these days. I really thought it'd be the exact opposite once I sold my practice. It may start with working out, a call with a client, replying to emails, or checking in on a rehab we have going. I like the variance and the fact that rarely does it include having to be some place at a certain time.

What is your biggest fear?

Losing a spouse or a child.

Please explain the most challenging time in your career and how you moved past it and thrived on the other side?

In 2009, I was still pretty young and naïve. I purchased a second practice. I didn't plan to work it; I was just going to own it, have an associate, and print money, right?

Well, it didn't work that way. I did not lead that practice like I should have, or now know how to. It was 100% my fault! Eventually the second practice was costing me over $10K a month to keep afloat. Thankfully, my first practice could handle it, but I was robbing Peter to pay Paul every month.

I finally got to the point where I said, "If this practice is going down, it's going down with me at the helm." So I sold my original practice, which had grown, and jumped into my second practice that was doing everything BUT growing.

I went in the practice and basically started from scratch. I'd prepare handouts for my team, and we'd train for a day each and every week in the beginning. We covered everything…phone skills, how to build rapport, how to discuss treatment, things to say, ways to act, etc. Eventually, these things began to be second nature for my team, and the practice started growing quickly. It was 2011 when I started full time (3 days a week) at my second practice, and thankfully, it doubled several times before I sold it in 2017.

Hands-down the best learning experience of my career on multiple levels.

What is your goal-setting process?

I write down the goals I want to accomplish after I've scrubbed the list against the overall vision I have for my life...I then place them in strategic places where I have to look at them several times a day.

What is the best investment you have made either inside your career or outside of dentistry?

I think there are so many different ways to answer this question, depending on how we're measuring "best". I'm going to go through some different "good" investments I've made. Not in a specific order:

1   **Hiring a coach EARLY in my career.** Coaching above all else helped to get my mindset in the right place. It helped me break through the limitations and glass ceilings I had in my life. It's when I internalized the fact that I could create my own destiny, and I wasn't limited to, or confined by, what others were doing or had done.

2   **Passive income streams.** I looked ahead in my life and realized that if my end game was to be financially free by age 40, it would be much easier to do that by having a certain amount of passive income coming in each and every month, as opposed to saving up some ungodly amount and dipping into that principal each month.

3   **Time with my family.** This kind of goes hand-in-hand with #2. I've purposefully done my best to design my life both while I was practicing dentistry, and since, to allow maximum time with my family. It hasn't always been easy, especially when my intent---- were to never have to drive an old beater, or live in a van dow

the river in order to be able to do that. My game had to improve to fit my vision and goals. That all being said, the hard work has been well worth it; I feel that there is no better investment than pouring into my children. However, without #'s 1 and 2 above, it would have been a much more difficult task to achieve.

Looking back, what advice would you give yourself on the day of your dental school graduation?

Couple things:

Assume there is nothing off the table with your practice and life, just some things that require more effort to achieve. It all depends on how bad you want them. If the vision you have set is worth it, it makes all the work to achieve it inconsequential.

If you need help or a mentor, which definitely helps most us, get it early on. Find someone who has done what you want to do, and listen to them!

In your opinion, what separates the top 10% of dentists from the bottom 90%?

Proper mindset, and the willingness to work hard.

After every call I have with my clients, they get a list of action items. I have some who have them completed in a week, and some that show up to the next call a month later with only half completed. Guess which ones are more successful? It's not rocket science.

What keeps struggling dentists struggling?

Excuses. Not focusing on the right things, or not putting the proper amount of effort into the right things. Poor leadership skills. Being afraid or too proud to ask for help. All of which can lead to a lack of confidence, and it's hard to have a thriving practice when you're not confident. Not arrogant...but confident.

What are the top 3 books every dental practice owner should read?

Rich Dad Poor Dad by Kiyosaki
Relentless by Tim Grover
The 10x Rule by Grant Cardone

If you had to narrow it down to a couple...what traits or skills do you think are most important in running an uncommonly successful practice?

Being relentless...which can be tough to explain in some ways. What I mean by that is being uncommonly successful is not easy, and it doesn't come with just rolling with the punches. You have to be willing to do things others won't, and you have to be willing to do them regardless of whether you "feel" like it most of the time.

All the people featured in this book are relentless in one way or another. They put in extraordinary amounts of effort and often sacrifice when most others wouldn't have.

It may mean giving up things you enjoy, especially in the beginning. Speaking only for myself, in the beginning of my practices and when starting The Lifestyle Practice, I couldn't count the number of times I had to pass on golfing with friends, stayed up late or woke up early while my family was sleeping so I wouldn't have to rob time from them, skipped social gatherings, spent time training my team when I'd rather be at home—and the list could go on. However, it all was a gamble I was willing to take. Now it has paid off and I have the time and finances at a relatively young age to live the life I want to live.

What is a skill or procedure you've added since graduating from dental school that has had a major positive impact on your practice?

As far as a skill, I would say leadership. Without leadership skills, our practice culture and ultimately my success would have been severely limited. Your practice will never outperform your level of leadership. If your leadership level is a 5, your practice is not going to be a 10.

A John Maxwell quote says, "He who thinks he leads, and has no one following him, is merely taking a walk." I could have never done what I did without a wonderful team and patients to support, trust, and follow.

As far as procedures, I would have to say implants and clear aligner therapy. Perhaps because those were the main elective treatments I performed, and even those were on a somewhat limited basis. If I were to start over, I would focus heavily on becoming skilled and efficient at selling and placing implants to help my patients.

What is the best business advice you ever received?

A few really jump out at me.

During my first couple years of college, I wasn't really sure what I was going to do when I grew up. I was not thrilled about the idea of going to school for 8 years until I was 26, and had some jealousy of my friends who knew they were only going to get a 4-year degree and then get out and start making some "real money". My mom had a come-to-Jesus talk with me and basically said, "You're going to be 26 someday either way. You can stop school early and work hard the rest of your life, or keep going and have an extraordinary life." Granted there were a few liberties and assumptions made in that talk, but I'm not sure where I'd be without it. That's a lot of wisdom coming from a woman who worked 32 years in a General Motors factory!

Another came from Bill Blatchford, and I'll never forget when he told me, "Be careful grabbing for brass rings." He had seen doctors get in trouble once they were making some grip investing in the newest and shiniest thing or idea. I've always heard that advice in the back of my mind whenever I evaluate different opportunities. It's helped me always remember that keeping the capital you make is as important as creating the capital itself.

What leadership advice would you give a dentist who has an ineffective culture in their practice?

Internalize that it all starts with YOU. How you do anything is how you do everything. If you need help, which most of us do, get it. Attend conferences, get a coach, read books on the subject. Don't be penny wise and a pound foolish when it comes to acquiring help to improve this skill!

What advice would you give a dentist that is struggling with case acceptance?

A lot! Understand case acceptance is a process that begins long before you enter the room to do your exam. Practice, practice...then practice some more. Read books on sales. Get help if needed.

What marketing advice would you give a dentist that is starting out in practice ownership?

Internalize and embrace that everything you do is marketing. Remember if you fail to differentiate, you will fail to attract. Analyze your different ROIs and continually refine your material. Have a good internal marketing plan in addition to external, and never forget the more the ACTION you take, the more results you will see.

What do our dental patients most desire?

Our patients most desire, what THEY desire. Find out what they want, and then give it to them. For some it may be a perfect smile, relationship, efficiency, getting out of pain, etc. You have to ask the right questions to figure this out, and when you do, focus on it and give it to them!

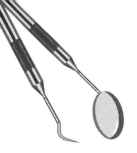

DR. BILL DORFMAN

Cosmetic Dentist, Extreme Makeover, The Doctors

Justin: *I actually was able to do this first interview with Dr. Dorfman on the phone. We had a great conversation, and it was clear to see, based off Bill's mindset and outlook on the world, why he has had such a successful career.*

Background

Dr. Bill Dorfman graduated from the University of the Pacific School of Dentistry in 1983. He has maintained one of the most successful aesthetic practices in the Beverly Hills, where he has created smiles for some of Hollywood's top stars including Usher, Jessica Simpson, The Osbournes, Hugh Jackman, Eva Longoria, Anthony Hopkins, Katy Perry, Fergie, and many others.

Dr. Bill was the founder of Discus Dental and is the author of *The Smile Guide* and NYT's bestseller *Billion Dollar Smile*. He frequently appears on national television, most recently appearing on *Oprah, Dr. Phil, The View, Larry King Live, Extreme Makeover,* and *The Doctors*.

In addition he has helped raise over 40 million dollars for children's hospitals and related charities with the Crown Council's

Smiles for Life campaign. He is also the founder of the non-profit LEAP foundation, a week-long summer motivational/leadership program for students 15–25 at UCLA, which just celebrated its 10-year anniversary.

Dr. Bill has already received 16 lifetime achievement awards and has recently been placed in the Guinness Book of World Records. Dr. Bill Dorfman has committed his life to the advancement of dentistry, philanthropy, health and fitness, and most importantly, his 3 daughters.

Please explain your style of practice (practice size, location, procedure mix, etc.)

I have a very unique FFS practice. I practice in a high-rise building between Hollywood and Beverly Hills. We take a lot of time with our patients; it's a very personalized practice.

We do a lot of cosmetic dentistry and we have the ability to custom stain and color our restorations. We have an in-office lab technician from DaVinci Dental. I practice part-time now hands-on and spend the rest of my time filming TV Shows and doing philanthropic work specifically with the Leap Foundation. [LeapFoundation.com]

Do you have a favorite success quote or mantra?

#1 – Don't wait for opportunities in life, make them.

#2 – When you get an opportunity, don't take it...master it!

In regards to your dental career, what would you like your legacy to be, or how would you like to be remembered?

I've had a unique career, but I think the thing I'm most proud of is the work I did with the Crown Council in raising over 40M dollars for Children's Charities in the Smile for Life Program.

What does success mean to you?

Success means not only achieving goals, but doing something meaningful. Not just meaningful for me, but something that also has a positive social impact on those around me.

What is your morning routine (first 1–2 hrs of the day)?

I am routine! The first thing I do is wake and say, "WIN"...which stands for What's Important Now. I literally and mentally go through my day and think about what are the important things I need to do. The next thing I do is I go and I have a protein smoothie; I've had the same protein smoothie for the last 35 years. Then I read the newspaper cover to cover.

Please explain the most challenging time in your career and how you moved past it and thrived on the other side?

The most challenging time in my career was in 2007. It was really weird; in April of the year, I remember driving to work and being so overwhelmed with the beauty around me, and I actually pulled over to the side of the road and had to stop just be appreciative and thankful. My kids were healthy, I was recently remarried, and we were on the verge of selling Discus Dental. Everything was really firing on all cylinders.

Then just a few months later in July, it all fell apart. My marriage started to fail, one of my close family members became really ill, and the sale of our company was aborted. It was a really tough time for me.

What is your goal-setting process?

It's pretty simple...if I think it, I can achieve it. The second part of this is...I refuse to fail. I never fail, because it's a mindset. If I try something and it doesn't work, I practice. If it doesn't work again, I practice some more, and sometimes I have to practice a lot. But you only really fail if you give up, and I refuse to give up. It's not that I never fail, I just never give up.

What is the best investment you have made either inside your career or outside of dentistry?

I feel like you have to answer that in two arenas. I honestly feel my best investment I ever made is in my kids. That ranks above and beyond everything else in your life. Being a parent and being present, loving, and supportive—that's the greatest investment I think any of us could ever give.

From a strictly business standpoint, I'd say we started Discus Dental from nothing. It was 3 guys and we were broke. And from nothing, we grew that company to $1.3 billion in sales.

Looking back, what advice would you give yourself on the day of your dental school graduation?

It's the same advice I've given at many keynotes and graduations, and it's the same advice I've given those students, and it's the same advice I'd give myself. As far as dentistry is concerned, graduating dental school and becoming a dentist is just the beginning.

I've used dentistry as a platform to do so many different things. You don't have to just sit in your office and drill teeth your entire career, unless that's what you want to do. For me, dentistry was a stepping stone to do things like being on primetime TV, being a NYT's best selling author, starting a successful dental company, and then founding an essential non-profit foundation in the Leap Foundation.

In your opinion, what separates the top 10% of dentists from the bottom 90%?

I think the thing that separates dentists is confidence. A lot of dentists just don't have any confidence, and your patients feel and sense that. When patients come to my practice and they're trusting me to be their dentist to improve their oral health or cosmetics, there has to be a level of trust.

If you don't have confidence in yourself, you don't exude that to your patients; and I think that's a big differentiator.

What keeps struggling dentists struggling?

They're not out perfecting their art. You can never stop learning. When I sit back and look at what I do on a day-to-day basis in my practice, over 90% of what I do I didn't learn in dental school. If your learning stops after dental school, you've become outdated right away. Dentists need to take courses, take CE, and never stop learning.

What are the top 3 books every dental practice owner should read?

Grit by Angela Duckworth
Think and Grow Rich by Napoleon Hill
The Tipping Point by Malcolm Gladwell

Dave: *I don't think it's a coincidence that the 3 books mentioned by one of dentistry's most renowned clinicians all have their foundation in mindset.*

If you had to narrow it down to a couple...what traits or skills do you think are most important in running an uncommonly successful practice?

People skills! The hardest part of business is actually dealing with your employees, not even our patients. Unfortunately, they don't teach that in school; but that's the hardest part. Cultivating and creating a culture, maintaining that culture, giving your employees a reason to stay and grow with you is the most difficult but most important skill we as dentists can have.

What is a skill or procedure you've added since graduating from dental school that has had a major positive impact on your practice?

For me, it is porcelain veneers. I'm applying for my third Guinness World Book record for doing more porcelain veneers than any dentist in the world. It's been a huge part of my practice.

What is the best business advice you ever received?

It was from my grandfather who was a mentor, and he said, "Make sure you sign every check," and, "No one cares about your money like you do."

What leadership advice would you give a dentist who has an ineffective culture in their practice?

First join the Crown Council; that's what it's all about. Also copy genius; go where people are doing a great job of doing this, learn what they do, and copy it.

Dave: *"Good artists copy. Great artists steal" —Pablo Picasso*

What advice would you give a dentist that is struggling with case acceptance?

One of the biggest problems I see dentists doing is being wishy-washy. You can offer people 25 treatment plans and confuse them. I don't do that. I basically sit down and tell them, "I've been practicing for 34 years; if your mouth were my mouth, this is what I'd do."

If they say, "That sounds like a great plan, but I don't have the financial resources to do that," then I have my office manager come in and figure out what we can do with what they have. I don't give my patients multiple treatment plans.

Justin: *This was one of my favorite answers in the entire book. A recurring theme you'll hear repeated over and over in this book is that you* *have to have confidence when talking to patients. If you don't, they will smell it a mile away. Being wishy-washy is a sure sign that confidence is lacking.*

What marketing advice would you give a dentist that is starting out in practice ownership?

Look in your area, or another area, and find a dentist with a practice like yours, with similar demographics, and copy what they do and improve on what they do.

What do our dental patients most desire?

What my patients want are beautiful, natural-looking smiles. Patients want it to look like they were just born with beautiful, natural teeth.

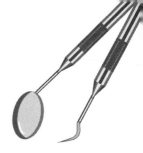

DR. PETER BOWMAN

Bowman Dental

Background

Born and raised in CA to lower-class and then later middle-class income parents.

When I was 4, I visited my grandparents after they rebuilt his (grandfather's) grandmother's house in Walpole, NH—a house that had been in his family for 3 generations prior. The house was massive and elegant, and VERY impressive to a 4-year-old (impressive to anyone, really). My grandfather told me that I could one day have a house like that, if I was willing to do what was necessary to have the money to afford it—which meant choosing a job that earned enough money and actually being willing to DO what's necessary. This was my first goal I ever had in life. At the time I had no idea what I wanted to do for a living. My grandfather used to tell many stories of HIS father, who was the area dentist and was a "doer" for the community. He got things done and he was well-respected. He made good money; however, he spent every dime he earned and he died broke. My grandfather taught me at a young age the importance of making a good income and saving it. And one day I'd be able to have a house like he did.

After dental school, I moved to Walpole to practice dentistry and be closer to my grandparents and with the intention of one day carrying the responsibilities to care for the house, which has now been enjoyed by 7 straight generations. My grandfather recently passed away from Alzheimer's. When my grandmother passes on and the house becomes empty, we will purchase it from the family estate so the family can continue to enjoy it.

Please explain your style of practice (practice size, location, procedure mix, etc.)

Small town; FFS and Delta Premier; Walpole, NH. General Dentistry and implants and bone grafting is a small portion of our production. Recently hired FT associate. Assisted hygiene schedule, 14 hygiene days a week.

Do you have a favorite success quote or mantra?

You Become What You Think About.

In regards to your dental career, what would you like your legacy to be, or how would you like to be remembered?

To be remembered as a good father, husband, neighbor, and friend. Remembered as an honest clinician who served the community better than any other dentist. Also to be known as someone who lived abundantly and happily and donated time and money abundantly back to the community who fueled my success. One who brought new ideas to the community that expand the mindsets and abundance to those who chose to be involved.

What does success mean to you?

"Success is the progressive realization of a worthy ideal."

—EARL NIGHTINGALE

What is your morning routine (first 1–2 hrs of the day)?

Wake up, shower, get dressed, make coffee and breakfast, read while eating, brush teeth, relax and often meditate for 5 minutes, kiss wife and kids good-bye, and leave for work. About meditation: I meditate by envisioning the things I want or want to be/do. At work: review every patient scheduled for the day for their treatment needs and unique needs, discuss them with the team at the morning huddle.

What is your biggest fear?

I've never been able to answer that question well and I've asked myself the question many times. Losing my family.

Please explain the most challenging time in your career and how you moved past it and thrived on the other side?

Taking a leap of faith to buy a small practice in my dream town with only 1 year of dental experience. To be honest, it never felt THAT challenging because I had full confidence that the decision was right. Other examples were when we decided to relocate/expand from 3 chairs to 8 chairs and invest $750,000 in building costs. We paid the debt off in less than 3 years. Again, it never felt like a challenge, because I was confident the rewards would be massive.

What is your goal-setting process?

Define them with specificity and with a deadline. Write them down. Recite them mentally or verbally IN THE FIRST-PERSON, PRESENT TENSE, on a daily basis until they become "common knowledge" to your brain, like second nature. I picture myself having accomplished the goal, and I generate the emotions and confidence I feel having accomplished them while I meditate.

What is the best investment you have made either inside your career or outside of dentistry?

My best investment was marrying my wife. Next best investments were becoming a dentist and owning a practice in a town where the dentistry was needed.

Looking back, what advice would you give yourself on the day of your dental school graduation?

Nothing. I was the last person accepted into my class. I had been given the gift of a lifetime and I wasn't about to lose it, nor complain about "how difficult and unfair dental school is".

In your opinion, what separates the top 10% of dentists from the bottom 90%?

The Top 10% think about what they want and how to get it. The Bottom 90% think about what they don't want, and who to blame.

Dave: *Peter draws a line in the sand. Winners vs. Whiners.*

What keeps struggling dentists struggling?

Mindset. A feeling of being trapped and helpless, whether they like dentistry or not. I argue they are not thinking about the right things; they're thinking about scarcity, fear, etc., rather than thinking about what they DO want in life and how dentistry can be the vehicle to achieving those things.

What are the top 3 books every dental practice owner should read?

The New Psychology of Achievement by Brian Tracy
Think and Grow Rich by Napoleon Hill
The Power of the Subconscious Mind by Joseph Murphy

Dave: I've known Peter for several years. We've had more than a few spirited discussions about classic texts like these and the psychology of success as a whole. You can tell by now that he's dedicated to mastery of his mindset.

If you had to narrow it down to a couple...what traits or skills do you think are most important in running an uncommonly successful practice?

Curiosity and eagerness. Never become content with what you have and what you do. Always find an interest and curiosity to expand into. This way you'll never be bored and eager to get out of dentistry.

What is a skill or procedure you've added since graduating from dental school that has had a major positive impact on your practice?

Time management. Always look for more efficient ways to achieve the same or higher results and quality. Clinically: implants and removable prosthodontics.

What is the best business advice you ever received?

Don't Lose Money!

What leadership advice would you give a dentist who has an ineffective culture in their practice?

First, understand yourself as well as you can. Be introspective. What are your strengths? Exploit them. What are your weaknesses? Seek out or hire others to help in those weaknesses. If you work harder at your weaknesses, you'll be left with some pretty strong weaknesses. Understand your personality and how you relate to others. Understand what environment and situations you perform best in (Conative qualities). Honestly assess your Emotional Intelligence and actively seek ways to continuously improve it.

Second, do the same for your team members. Teach them about their differences and how each person's strengths can be used to best serve the practice and their teammates. Get the people on the right seats in the bus.

Empower the team members to make decisions about what is best for the practice, and ask them to follow up and follow through with you about their decisions.

Be aware of qualities your team as a whole is missing, and when it's time to grow and expand the team, actively look for those with the qualities.

What advice would you give a dentist that is struggling with case acceptance?

Ask yourself, "What is it about ME that I can improve? Is it my personality? Am I too technical? Can I relate to the patient?" Seek out communication courses and practice the teachings until they become second nature to you.

What do our dental patients most desire?

Trust in receiving honest and quality and positive experiences with their dental office.

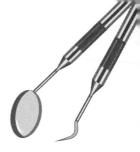

DR. GINA DORFMAN

Dentistry for Kids and Adults, Creator of YAPI

Background

I was born in St. Petersburg, Russia. I came to the United States with my dad in 1989, just after I finished 9th grade. After taking some placement tests, I was able to start community college, taking mostly ESL courses and science.

I considered a career in medicine, but dentistry seemed like a better fit because I always wanted to own my business, and it seemed that dentistry offered a more streamlined path to business ownership.

While in college, I worked in a few dental practices, starting as a filing clerk and eventually managing a large multi-location practice. I've seen a lot of different styles of practice. By the time I started dental school, I had a pretty good idea what my practice would be like one day.

I graduated from USC Dental School in 2000 and started my dental practice from scratch in 2002.

Being in a very competitive environment, I knew that the only way I could be successful is by being efficient. I also believed that if I had good office systems, I could hire smart people with great attitude and train them easily. I became obsessed with creating simple, reproducible systems. I've created, implemented, tweaked, and revised my systems until I felt I was able to eliminate any unnecessary steps and simplify everything else. I wanted to build a paperless ecosystem, improve communication, automate repetitive tasks, and organize office workflows. In the process, I've come up with a long list of things that I wished my practice management software could do. Eventually, I turned to my dad, a veteran software engineer, for help. My dad had just recently retired and was already showing the signs of boredom.

As I shared my ideas, he asked a lot of his usual "What's the point?" questions. The next morning, he showed me something that would turn out to be our next business venture. YAPI began as a simple intra-office communication software. As we implemented YAPI in my practice, my team and I began to come up with more ideas, and my dad never looked bored again. I showed YAPI to a few friends and they loved it. One of them posted about YAPI on DentalTown. The response was overwhelming. In 2011, we introduced YAPI at the Townie meeting in Las Vegas and signed our first 11 customers. By the end of our first year, we had 75 customers. Building a software company was a great adventure that allowed me to travel, meet a lot of great people, and work with my family. Now, 6 years later, we have over 30 employees, thousands of customers, and big development plans for the future.

Please explain your style of practice (practice size, location, procedure mix, etc.)

Dentistry for Kids and Adults is a family practice. With a team of 3 general dentists and 2 specialists, we are able to offer care to everyone in the family: from baby teeth to wisdom teeth, all under one roof. Often, new patients come in and have such a pleasant experience with us that they bring their children to our office, and later refer their parents. And when the children grow up, they bring their kids.

Seeing generations of families, getting to know them, and being there to help and be a part of their lives year after year is what still gets me out of bed in the morning excited to come to work.

When I come to the office, I am surrounded by smiling, happy people. I love walking through the office and watching my employees interact with patients, hearing friendly conversations and laughter. I don't know who said, "Surround yourself with positive people," but it's been my hiring philosophy ever since I've started my practice. I often joke with my team that our practice IS The Happiest Place on Earth. Everyone here loves what they do, and they genuinely like other people. This is not to say that they don't work hard or don't have bad days. Bad days happen, but we know how to pull together and remember to have fun.

Do you have a favorite success quote or mantra?

I just saw a quote by Zig Ziglar that Karah Maloley posted on Facebook: "You don't build a business, you build people, and people build a business." This makes so much sense to me. I haven't heard this quote until recently, but I've always operated this way. I always felt that my job as a business owner is to seek out bright people, identify their strengths, and help them build on these strengths.

I have so many talented, loyal, and hardworking employees in both my software company and my dental practice who contribute ideas, innovation, and passion every day. Every bit of success that I've enjoyed is because of these contributions.

In regards to your dental career, what would you like your legacy to be, or how would you like to be remembered?

I never thought about "my legacy" before. My mother-in-law always says, "It's better to give with warm hands." It means, it's better to give while you are alive, so that you could see the benefit of the gift. While the expression is about monetary gifts, I think it can apply to ideas as well as material things. I'd like to be remembered as a go-giver, someone who shared ideas freely and enjoyed seeing others benefit from them.

Dave: *Having known Gina for several years, I can attest to her generosity. It doesn't matter if it's leadership wisdom, a compliment, or something more tangible...Gina always gives more than she takes.*

What does success mean to you?

Success is waking up in the morning with a smile, eager to make the day count, and going to bed satisfied that I've made a difference, did my best, and stayed true to my values.

What is your morning routine (first 1–2 hrs of the day)?

I am a mom of 2 school-age kids. My morning routine is rather hectic. Once the kids are off to school, I usually get ready for work if I am seeing patients or go on a hike and listen to an audio book. I prefer business books. When I get home, I spend the next few hours working on my most important project. Then, I check my email, Facebook, Dentaltown, and Slack and catch up on the small things that need to be done.

What is your biggest fear?

My biggest fear is being blindsided by something that I either don't understand or cannot control.

Please explain the most challenging time in your career and how you moved past it and thrived on the other side?

The most challenging part of my career is balancing home and work. I love my work, and I love working, but I also want to make sure that I am there for my kids and that I don't miss anything. It takes a lot of planning, logistics, and discipline to keep it all together. Most of the time I feel like I have everything under control and then I realize that I forgot something. LOL

What is your goal-setting process?

I like to envision what it's going to look like when a specific goal is accomplished and reverse engineer the steps from there. I find that often, by the time I reach my goal, I already have a new goal in mind.

What is the best investment you have made either inside your career or outside of dentistry?

I feel that building a team that can carry on even when I am not around and building a practice that runs without me is by far the best investment I've made.

Looking back, what advice would you give yourself on the day of your dental school graduation?

Buy real estate.

In your opinion, what separates the top 10% of dentists from the bottom 90%?

The bottom 90% of the dentists will come up with a million reasons WHY something CANNOT be done. The successful 10% will instead question, "HOW CAN we do it?"

What keeps struggling dentists struggling?

It reminds me of a quote from Tolstoy's Anna Karenina: "Happy families are all alike; every unhappy family is unhappy in its own way." The same with dentists. All successful dentists have the same key qualities that help them succeed. All struggling dentists struggle for different reasons.

For some it's the mindset. They don't see success as a possibility. They blame the DSOs and the HMOs and they don't take ownership of the struggle. For others, it's simply the lack of business management skills or leadership skills. Some keep doing the same thing expecting different results. Others try a lot of different things but they don't think them through and don't stick with anything. In general, dentists are notorious for not training their teams well. Whether they don't want to close the office for training or worry that an employee will get training and leave, they simply don't invest into their team.

What are the top 3 books every dental practice owner should read?

The Pumpkin Plan by Mike Michalowicz
Leaders Eat Last by Simon Sinek
Drive by Daniel Pink

If you had to narrow it down to a couple...what traits or skills do you think are most important in running an uncommonly successful practice?

Passion. Willingness to push outside of the comfort zone. Narrow focus. Persistence. Commitment to continuous improvement. Great verbal skills and even better listening skills.

What is a skill or procedure you've added since graduating from dental school that has had a major positive impact on your practice?

Verbal skills.

What is the best business advice you ever received?

Instead of being all things to all people, figure out your ideal customer and build your business around this customer.

What leadership advice would you give a dentist who has an ineffective culture in their practice?

Culture can make or break a practice. Take a few days away from the practice. Go somewhere where you feel inspired and think about the kind of a practice you'd like to run one day. Think about your core values, your employees, your patients. Create a vivid Painted Picture of what your practice will look like 3 years from now. Go back to your team and communicate your Painted Picture, your values, and your mission to the team. Show them how they fit into that picture. Communicate frequently. Hire people who are excited about your Painted Picture and want to be a part of it.

Once you find out that someone is a great culture fit, treat them right and do everything in your power to retain them and help them grow. Don't hesitate to let go of people who don't fit into your culture or don't evolve with it. Lastly, keep in mind that creating a company culture takes work and it's not something that will just stay the same once you create it—it needs to be nurtured continuously.

Dave: *Every organization has a culture. Either by design or default. The default cultures are not generally healthy ones, so we should heed Gina's advice and define the ideal practice we want to work in.*

What advice would you give a dentist that is struggling with case acceptance?

George Bernard Shaw said, "The single biggest problem in communication is the illusion that it has taken place." Poor communication leads to lack of trust and lack of trust leads to poor case acceptance. Using an intra-oral camera is very helpful. Using good verbal skills is important. Teaching our assistants and hygienists to participate in co-diagnosis is critical. Good hand-off from back to front is also important.

But the most important thing we can do to increase case acceptance is to make sure that our patients understand and own the problem before you start offering your solutions. Too often, we quickly diagnose a problem, come up with a treatment plan and start "selling" our treatment plan to a patient who is not aware of a problem. This is when the patient will often ask: "How long can I wait?" What the patient is really saying is, "How long before I will experience a problem and will have to do this?" Instead of jumping into solutions, take a few minutes to explain the problem. Pull up a digital x-ray or an intra-oral image. Explain what you see in plain words. Better yet, use Socratic method to lead the patient in discovering the problem. When a patient asks, "Can you fix it?" you know they are ready to hear your solutions.

What marketing advice would you give a dentist that is starting out in practice ownership?

Find your niche—your uniqueness. Figure out who your ideal patients are, who can benefit the most from your unique offering. Create your marketing to attract your ideal patients.

What do our dental patients most desire?

Honesty. They want to know that their healthcare providers genuinely care about them and can be trusted.

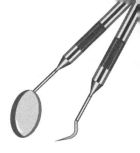

DR. ARUN GARG

Centers for Dental Implants, Implant Seminars

Background

Dr. Arun K. Garg is a nationally recognized dental educator and surgeon who for over 20 years served as a full-time professor of surgery in the division of oral and maxillofacial surgery and as director of residency training at the University of Miami Leonard M. Miller school of medicine. Frequently awarded faculty member of the year by his residents, Dr. Garg is considered the world's preeminent authority on bone biology, bone harvesting, and bone grafting for dental implant surgery and has written and published a dozen books and related surgical manuals, along with a dental implant marketing kit that has been translated in multiple languages and distributed worldwide.

He has been a featured speaker at dozens of state, national, and international dental association conventions and meetings including the American Academy of Periodontology, the American College of Oral and Maxillofacial Surgeons, and the International Dental Implant Associations. Dr. Garg earned his engineering degree from the University of Florida and completed his residency training at the University of Miami Jackson Memorial Hospital. He is also the founder of Implant Seminars, a leader in postgraduate dental implant continuing education, a company that offers a variety of hands-on and lecture-based courses.

Dave: *I did my early implant training with Dr. Garg. Between a 4-week-end continuum in Seattle and the hands-on training in the Dominican Republic, it gave me all the confidence I needed to start choosing the right cases and implementing the procedure in my practice.*

Please explain your style of practice (practice size, location, procedure mix, etc.)

I own several practices throughout South Florida and each one has been strategically located to cater to the unique demographics of the specified area. Practice size varies, as does procedure mix. For instance, in more affluent areas, there's a focus on more elective cosmetic surgeries and dental implants. In more working class areas, the focus is on basic maintenance and stressing the value of re-care visits.

Do you have a favorite success quote or mantra?

In my marketing book *Implant Excellence*, I often reference the imagination, determination, and efficiency of Walt Disney—about how he appreciated that the ride was only one part of the Disney experience.

From the moment guests walked into the park to the moment they left, they existed in Disney's world. Thus, for Disney, dreams and hard work went hand in hand.

Two of his quotes come to mind: "If you can dream it, you can do it." "The way to get started is to quit talking and begin doing."

Justin: *There are several great biographies written on Walt Disney, and I've always found him a great inspiration for thinking outside the box while building your business.*

In regards to your dental career, what would you like your legacy to be, or how would you like to be remembered?

At the core, dentists are healers—men and women who find genuine satisfaction in restoring health or physical beauty to the people we treat. With a complete appreciation of humility and, to borrow from the late astronomer and educator Carl Sagan, a full understanding of human fallibility, I would like to be most remembered for my work as a pioneer in bone biology, in the frontier work I did in discovering the applications of platelet-rich plasma to dentistry, and of course, as an educator who worked tirelessly to empower students with the same knowledge I possess.

What does success mean to you?

Success is relative to the individual. But for me, it means a combination of material comfort, the genuine pleasure I feel in helping the patients I treat, and educating thousands of dentists since I began the earliest version of what would become Implant Seminars more than 30 years ago.

Dave: *It seems simple, but I think it's important to highlight that "success" is between you and you, as Dr. Garg mentions. Too often, we as dentists chase other people's dreams. Therefore, it's critically important for each of us to have a clear vision for what we want to give and get during our careers.*

What is your morning routine (first 1–2 hrs of the day)?

As the CEO and founder of a dental implant continuing education company, as well as the owner of several dental practices across South Florida, the first few hours of my day are spent reviewing emails from each area I oversee. That could mean following up with doctors who have specific questions related to material covered in my courses, patients inquiring about services, and also just follow-ups with staff and my office managers. I try to limit this first task of the day to 2 hours at most, as I have to prioritize my scheduling for my lecturing, surgeries, and prep time for both.

What is your biggest fear?

I wouldn't call it a fear. Just a nagging sense that there are always more people to educate. A teacher's work is never done. I also never want to let my family—or my patients—down. I say this in the same sentence because so many of my patients have become extensions of family.

Please explain the most challenging time in your career and how you moved past it and thrived on the other side?

I gave this question serious thought. In my experience, the transition from academia to private practice was one of my greatest professional hurdles. In academia, I had little patient interaction time, whereas in private practice, establishing those human connections was critical. I also had to learn how to become a marketing professional. They don't teach you that in dental school either. And you certainly don't get to practice that skill set teaching. So I had to spend considerable funds taking additional courses in these areas. It was a lot to learn in such a short timeframe.

Justin: In looking at Dr. Garg from an outsider's perspective, I know it's easy to think, of all people, surely Dr. Garg wouldn't struggle heading into private practice. I'm glad he shared this, because it's a good reminder that the ease of which something comes to us, isn't the determining factor of eventual success.

What is your goal-setting process?

I take the time to assess where I'm at professionally, what I have achieved, and what I expect to achieve in a certain timeframe. I then write down the concrete steps I'm taking to achieve those goals. I don't do this every day or even every week. But I can't stress enough how important it is to not only write down one's goals, but to itemize how they're being achieved or not. If it's not written down, it's not real.

What is the best investment you have made either inside your career or outside of dentistry?

Decades ago, one of my mentors stressed the importance of dental specialization. For me that was implantology. It's been a privilege helping pioneer the advancement of dental implants and educating fellow dentists on how to incorporate these treatments into their practice. It's transformed my life. It's transformed the lives of my students. And it's transformed the lives of the patients all of us treat.

Looking back, what advice would you give yourself on the day of your dental school graduation?

That's easy. To be open minded to new treatment-planning methodologies, to never stop learning, and to always embrace the business side of dentistry. Because it doesn't matter if you're the world's greatest dentist and nobody knows about it. You have to be skilled in promotion and marketing in order to acquire, engage, and retain patients.

In your opinion, what separates the top 10% of dentists from the bottom 90%?

This answer relates to the above question. The bottom 90% aren't poor clinicians—most of them, at least. They lack the marketing skills to get the word out. Many still think like academics. They haven't taken additional courses in business. They haven't broadened their skills since dental school. (For some, that could be decades ago.) And they haven't connected with patients in business-savvy ways that empower them to become your brand's biggest supporters and promoters.

Dave: *This reminds me of a quote that I read early on during my startup by marketing legend Dan Kennedy. It was a HUGE paradigm shift for me. I'll paraphrase to make it applicable to dentistry: "The most import-ant day in a dentist's life is when in his mind (s)he stops being a dentist and becomes a marketer of dental services."*

What keeps struggling dentists struggling?

Doing the same thing year after year and expecting different results. Dentists who are unwilling to learn or who are set in their ways face the greatest challenge. Obsolescence doesn't happen overnight. It's a process that begins so slowly you don't even notice it. It's like the frog in boiling water scenario. Increase the temperature instantly and the frog knows it's in danger. Raise the water temperature slowly and the frog will meet its demise. In my experience, struggling dentists aren't even fully aware of just how much they're struggling.

If you had to narrow it down to a couple...what traits or skills do you think are most important in running an uncommonly successful practice?

Confidence, marketing awareness, business management skills, flexibility, intelligence, the ability to see the bigger picture, and genuineness.

What is a skill or procedure you've added since graduating from dental school that has had a major positive impact on your practice?

Also an easy question. For me, that would be dental implantology and then augmenting basic implant skills with more advanced bone grafting treatment planning. Digital dentistry is also gaining a lot of traction these days, as is in-house milling.

What is the best business advice you ever received?

Don't pigeonhole yourself into any single specialty. Recognize the speed with which dentistry, dental technology, and patient desires are evolving. Meet those needs head on. And don't be afraid to fail.

What leadership advice would you give a dentist who has an ineffective culture in their practice?

Look inward first. Have that dentist perform an exercise and ask him or her to write down all of their character strengths and weaknesses. Or write out a list of declarative leadership statements and ask the dentist in question to grade themselves on a percentage scale. For instance: "I am a good motivator." Do you agree with this statement 50% of the time, 75%, or 100% all of the time? You could also hand out surveys asking the same questions to generate a more objective response.

What advice would you give a dentist that is struggling with case acceptance?

First is to quantify the struggle. You can't manage what you don't measure. How poor is your case acceptance really? Once you know exactly which patients turned down treatment, it wouldn't hurt to send an email or text follow-up. It's your mission to determine why they declined treatment. Once you learn these answers, you can improve your marketing efforts to satisfy those needs.

What marketing advice would you give a dentist that is starting out in practice ownership?

Search engine optimization and Google rank orderings are incredibly important. Work with a profession either outsourced or in-house who knows how to use the web to your marketing advantage. But at the same time, don't forget the value of traditional outreach. Nothing speaks like the voice of authenticity better than a patient singing your praise to a family member or friend.

What do our dental patients most desire?

The most affordable, most aesthetic, most comfortable restoration in the fastest and safest time possible.

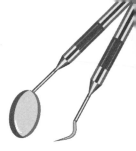

DR. BRAD STUTLER

Stutler Dental,
Transcend Dental Partners

Justin: *I met Brad at an event several years ago now. After getting to talk a bit over the weekend, I just really liked him. He runs an incredible practice in Indy. He was a great help and encouragement to me while I was beginning The Lifestyle Practice, and has a ton of knowledge to offer about running an incredible, high-performing dental practice. We're excited to share his story with you.*

Background

Graduated from Indiana University 2002. Started a scratch practice in 2005. The last twelve years have been a whirlwind. Personally, I have 3 kids that are 9, 7, and 5...definitely my most exciting accomplishment along with my awesome wife, Susie. Our dental office has continually performed in the top 1% nationally over the last decade, thanks to building a great team.

Currently I've started a DSO, Transcend Dental Partners. Our goal is to have 50 practices in the next 5 years.

Please explain your style of practice (practice size, location, procedure mix, etc.)

We have a fast-paced environment that focuses on amazing customer service while being efficient and profitable. Located in Brownsburg, Indiana (just outside of Indianapolis), we have 8 operatories and a team of 12. Procedurally, we keep most things in house, referring out only limited oral surgery, ortho, and endo.

Do you have a favorite success quote or mantra?

"Do or Do Not, There is NO Try!"

—YODA

*"If you get enough should's in life,
you'll should all over yourself."*

—TONY ROBBINS

In regards to your dental career, what would you like your legacy to be, or how would you like to be remembered?

Ultimately, I want to be remembered as someone who really cared about his team and his patients. Hopefully my team will look back and remember me as someone who not only invested in their dental education, but more importantly was investing in them to become better people.

Dave: *Investing in your team to make them better people is a powerful leadership lesson. Good for them, good for you. Good for your practice, community, and legacy!*

What does success mean to you?

Spending time with my family. I came from a household where my parents worked what seemed like 80 hours a week to ensure that my brother and I had the best opportunities. Being a great dad and husband is the best payback that I can give my parents who have sacrificed so much for my success.

What is your morning routine (first 1–2 hrs of the day)?

A typical day consists of getting up around 5am. Lifting weights for 45 minutes and some form of cardio for 20–30 minutes. Breakfast and out the door. And lots of coffee!!

What is your biggest fear?

Looking back and regretting not taking more chances in life. As Gary Vaynerchuk says, when asked how do you stay motivated, "I'm going to die!"

Dave: *Interesting that the #1 regret of the dying is nearly identical and also based in courage: "I wish I'd had the courage to live a life true to myself, not the life others expected of me."*

Please explain the most challenging time in your career and how you moved past it and thrived on the other side?

In 2013–14, I was seriously burnt out on dentistry. My office had become a monster, and I felt exhausted all of the time. I stepped back and looked at what I needed to do to regain control. By cutting my hours and adding an associate, I've been able to increase my profitability, and my personal life has thrived.

What is your goal-setting process?

I think of generalized goals first. Then pick my top 3–4 goals and narrow them down. Being specific and having clear timelines.

What is the best investment you have made either inside your career or outside of dentistry?

I still think that the best thing that I ever did before opening my practice in 2005 was reading and watching everything that I could find from Howard Farran. He along with Bruce Baird and Mike Abernathy have taught me more about business than any other source. Outside of dentistry, my wife and I recently invested in attending Tony Robbins UPW in NYC. The investment has really accelerated her AirBnB rental business. The bottom line is never stop investing in yourself! We are all either growing or dying!

Looking back, what advice would you give yourself on the day of your dental school graduation?

Think huge goals!! I think most of us have small goals that are way too easy. Thus, we then get bored. Looking back, I would have started multiple practices from day one.

In your opinion, what separates the top 10% of dentists from the bottom 90%?

Goals and FEAR. I believe that the top 10% in any profession or sport are ultra competitive and goal oriented. They have a clear vision, and they know their WHY. Unfortunately, our engineer personalities lend us to being very risk averse. Leading us to being hesitant in making decisions. Although I have fearful thoughts, I tell myself that is BS, and I keep moving forward toward my goals.

What keeps struggling dentists struggling?

Limiting beliefs!! If you think you can or can't, you are correct!

Justin: I couldn't agree more with Brad on this answer. Limiting beliefs are a silent killer in underperforming offices. Often seeing is believing, and I hope some of the stories in this book help in starting to erase those belief systems that can hold us back. If it's been done before, it can surely be done again!

What are the top 3 books every dental practice owner should read?

The Success Principles by Jack Canfield

How to Win Friends and Influence People by Carnegie

Emotional Intelligence 2.0 by Bradbury and Greaves

If you had to narrow it down to a couple...what traits or skills do you think are most important in running an uncommonly successful practice?

Communication skills—myself and my team are very clear communicators with our patients. Thus, we have high case acceptance. Personality profiling—whether it be DISC, Meyer-Briggs, etc. This greatly helps in understanding your patients and your team.

What is a skill or procedure you've added since graduating from dental school that has had a major positive impact on your practice?

Conscious sedation! This along with implants and CEREC have been wonderful additions. Patients that don't remember me seem to love me. I'm not sure what that says about my personality.

What is the best business advice you ever received?

You are a business owner that happens to be a dentist.

What leadership advice would you give a dentist who has an ineffective culture in their practice?

Get a coach! The most successful people in the world have coaches. More importantly, listen to them. There is a reason that the culture is ineffective, and usually it's the dentist.

Dave: *This has been a common theme with our Titans. They didn't hesitate to spend money on getting support from a coach and shortening the learning curve.*

What advice would you give a dentist that is struggling with case acceptance?

Get out your iphone or ipad and record your presentations. Although it will seem awkward at first, the amount of insight gained will be well worth it. Every sports team records their games and practices. Why? They go back through the tape and figure out how could they get better. Then compare yourself to the masters like Bruce Baird.

What marketing advice would you give a dentist that is starting out in practice ownership?

Never stop marketing! Always remember, 50% of the population does not go to the dentist on a regular basis. That way, you can establish a brand and be first in the consumer's mind when you are needed. We religiously spend 5–7% on marketing.

Justin: *Again another top performing office, making a sizable investment in marketing month after month, even after the practice is doing very well.*

What do our dental patients most desire?

Health and to be heard. The days of dictating treatment is long gone. Listening to the patient will allow us to be ultra successful.

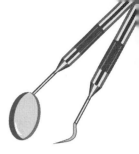

DR. GORDON J. CHRISTENSEN

Prosthodontist, Practical Clinical Courses, Clinicians Report Foundation

Background

Gordon J. Christensen is Founder and Chief Executive Officer of Practical Clinical Courses (PCC), Chief Executive Officer of Clinicians Report Foundation (CR), and a practicing Prosthodontist in Provo, Utah.

Gordon and Dr. Rella Christensen are co-founders of the non-profit Clinicians Report Foundation (previously named CRA). Currently, Dr. Rella Christensen is the Director of the TRAC Research Division of the CR Foundation. Since 1976, they have conducted research in all areas of dentistry and published the findings to the profession in the well-known CRA Newsletter now called *Clinicians Report*.

Gordon's degrees include: DDS, University of Southern California; MSD, University of Washington; PhD, University of Denver; and two honorary doctorates.

Early in his career, Gordon helped initiate the University of Kentucky and University of Colorado dental schools and taught at the University of Washington.

Currently, he is an Adjunct Professor at the University of Utah, School of Dentistry. Gordon has presented thousands of hours of continuing education globally, made hundreds of educational videos used throughout the world, and published widely.

Gordon and Rella's sons are dentists. William is a prosthodontist, and Michael is a general dentist. Their daughter, Carlene, is an administrator in a biomedical company.

He is a member of numerous professional organizations.

Please explain your style of practice (practice size, location, procedure mix, etc.)

Multi operatory eclectic practice in Provo, Utah. Mainly the complete realm of prosthodontics, plus everything else in dentistry, since we do research in all areas of dentistry.

Do you have a favorite success quote or mantra?

YOU CAN DO IT
DO IT NOW
IT WILL ALL WORK OUT

In regards to your dental career, what would you like your legacy to be, or how would you like to be remembered?

Educator, researcher, practitioner, altruistic person. Co-Founder of Clinical Research Associates, now named Clinician's Report.

What does success mean to you?

Satisfaction and enjoyment in every area of life.
Honest service to people.
Adequate financials to fund family needs.

What is your morning routine (first 1–2 hrs of the day)?

Up at 4am.

5am to office or wherever I am working on a given day to practice, research organization, courses, or church work.

What is your biggest fear?

I have no major fears, and as I said, it will all work out. There is a higher power guiding me.

Please explain the most challenging time in your career and how you moved past it and thrived on the other side?

I had about 15 years of full-time academics, but I realized I had more potential.

I started our research and educational organizations in spite of colleagues telling me private non-profit research and private education would not work. We are now enjoying 41 years of success.

What is your goal-setting process?

Annual planning retreat.
Quarterly planning retreat.
Monthly planning retreat.
Weekly follow-up on goals.
Daily follow-up on goals.

What is the best investment you have made either inside your career or outside of dentistry?

Pertaining to financial investments...a few real estate deals.
My best investment overall was going to dental school.

Looking back, what advice would you give yourself on the day of your dental school graduation?

To do exactly what I have done. Be your own boss.

In your opinion, what separates the top 10% of dentists from the bottom 90%?

Optimism, enthusiasm, drive, creativity, leadership.

A passion for dentistry. An eclectic lifestyle.

Learning some significant new procedure or concept each year and implementing it into life.

Dave: *Changing up the procedure mix is a great way to keep variety in the practice for the doctor and team, better serving our patients, and a way to keep the practice revenues growing each year. Innovation is a great way to differentiate yourself from the other dental offices in your community, since most dentists are adding new skill sets or technology on a regular basis.*

What keeps struggling dentists struggling?

Lack of what I mentioned in the last question.

I disdain the phrase some dentists state when asked how it's going and they say, "Same ol', same ol'."

What are the top 3 books every dental practice owner should read?

Good to Great by Jim Collins
Flip Your Focus by Bob Spiel
Team of Teams by Gen. McChrystal

If you had to narrow it down to a couple...what traits or skills do you think are most important in running an uncommonly successful practice?

Leadership, organization, empathy for staff, excellent staff salaries, delegation of all legal tasks to staff. Multiple operatory practice, constant CE, constant communication with staff, bonus for specific tasks. Praise when deserved.

Dave: *Dr. Christiansen is one of the most influential clinicians of our time, but he points out that solid leadership is the core of an uncommonly successful practice. That's powerful!*

What is a skill or procedure you've added since graduating from dental school that has had a major positive impact on your practice?

Implant placement. Lots of technology. Veneers. All of esthetic dentistry. Hypnosis.

What is the best business advice you ever received?

Buy things when you have the money. Adjust your practice to the needs of your patients, not the reverse. Be absolutely honest. Don't do anything to the patient you would not do to yourself.

What leadership advice would you give a dentist who has an ineffective culture in their practice?

Staff meetings monthly.
Huddles daily.
Staff parties.
Staff bonuses.
Constant CE.
Excellent pay for staff.
Opportunities for staff to enhance their skills and knowledge.

What advice would you give a dentist that is struggling with case acceptance?

Implement a staff-oriented diagnostic data-collection appointment.
Use teaching aids, models, videos, handouts, etc.

What marketing advice would you give a dentist that is starting out in practice ownership?

Use patient testimonials to influence other patients.
Don't advertise overtly in the media.
Use educational info in your practice.
Reward patients who refer to you.
Don't self promote.
Be fair with patients financially.

What do our dental patients most desire?

Honest treatment plans.
Moderate fees.
Conservative dentistry.

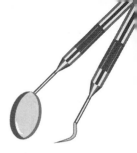

DR. ERIN ELLIOTT

Post Falls Family Dental,
Past President of American Sleep
and Breathing Academy

Background

I grew up down in Southern California, Orange County, and decided that there was life outside of California, and went to undergrad, a small Christian school called Houghton College in Houghton, New York, on a soccer and athletic scholarship. The reason why I chose that school versus UCLA—where I was born and raised to go, strived to go, and accepted to—was because at that time, I was looking for an adventure.

I was seeking an opportunity to be a scholar athlete, but at Houghton, it's where I discovered that I could actually be an athlete and a scholar. Grades were really important to me. Therefore, if I had to miss a practice in order to go to science lab so that I could actually be a biology major, then I would not be penalized.

I met my husband there. Got married after my junior year of undergrad, and then got into Creighton University in Omaha, NE for dental school. I decided to look at private colleges since I was no longer a California resident; my family had moved to Washington State, and

I wasn't a Washington State resident, and I wasn't really a New York resident as well. I was kind of stuck in this no-man's land and applied to different private schools and got in at Creighton.

I enjoyed my time there. I graduated in 2003, graduated fifth in my class, out of 5, (just kidding) out of 86. We then came and settled in Post Falls, Idaho, so that I could start a family and start in the practice that I found.

Please explain your style of practice (practice size, location, procedure mix, etc.)

I practice in a town of 28,000. It is between Spokane, Washington and Coeur d'Alene, Idaho.

My county is pretty large, and it has about 100,000. We have a family dental practice in which we see patients 2 to 102. We have a large demographic of retired people here, as well as blue collar and white collar. It's an awesome place to live. We definitely celebrate the four seasons, and really focus on family.

We have a huge procedure mix. The only things we refer out are extreme cases. We do implants and refer out the more complicated ones, but we do have an associate here on Thursdays, a retired dentist, who does most of our surgeries as far as impacted wisdom teeth and sinus lifts, etc.

We do a lot of extractions and partials, implants, fillings. We really do have a huge mix. My next endeavor is going to be placing implants myself and taking implant pathways, so that I can do some of the bigger, more complicated cases.

We also treat a lot of sleep apnea, which is one of my specialties and expertise.

Do you have a favorite success quote or mantra?

I don't know if I have a favorite success quote or mantra, but one of my favorites is one that my Dad kind of imparted to me, because I'm such a nerd and I worked so hard in dental school. One thing I've learned, is that patients don't care how much you know, they just want to know how much you care.

And I think that is a huge thing in creating relationships. We have a really homey style practice, where we do know everybody's names, and we know their families, and we run into them in the community. We are a part of the community. I love kind of that small town feel that we have here.

The other quote that I really like—I saw it on a meme with Simon Sinek. I don't know if it's him that actually said it. But it says, "Working hard for something you don't care about is called stress. Working hard for something you love is called passion."

I feel like I am in an awesome place in life where I love my job, I love coming to work every day. There is stress, but it's just kind of all part of it. I will continue to work enthusiastically and passionately, because I love what we do, and at the root of it, I love being able to speak, as well, and travel, even though I hate public speaking.

That is because I want other dentists to feel the passion, and I want other dentists to love their job.

In regards to your dental career, what would you like your legacy to be, or how would you like to be remembered?

In regards to my legacy. I am only 40, so I don't know how much of a legacy I have yet, but let's say I died today. I think at my funeral what they would say about me is that—is how passionate I was about, and how much enthusiasm I had, for people and for my job. To see them get better, to see them smile, to see them sleep. I really think that they would talk about my energy and my passion.

I think dentistry kind of oozes out of my pores. In fact, when my kids do an impersonation of me, this is kind of funny. This is the quote. "I'm Erin, 'dental stuff'...Hey, I know you!" That's because I am quite combined in dentistry and relationships.

What does success mean to you?

Obviously, success, to most people—and this probably sounds trite—is that it's not about the money. However, you will be profitable. You do need to make money in order to really show up every day. But success to me would be seeing my teen meet their personal goals, professionally as well as personally. Success means being happy and passionate about what you do. To not wake up in the morning and drag yourself out of bed.

What is your morning routine (first 1–2 hrs of the day)?

My morning routine is to wake-up at 5am, 10-till, because sometimes I press snooze. I listen to podcasts on my 20-minute drive to the gym. I get a workout in, and I really don't love cardio. I do cardio, but it's usually as I'm listening to a podcast or being able to read a book, so I'm usually on the elliptical or the bike.

Hit the shower, and I'm at work around 6:45. We start the day out with a morning huddle. I'm usually one of the first to be here. I think it sets a good example, but it's also so that I can be prepared for the day.

End that morning huddle, and then we start our patients at 7:10. Even when I'm on vacation, I really miss my routine. I think there is something to be said about the early bird catches the worm. Most successful people I know do get up early. There are times I do morning meetings at 6am, if people are willing to meet me at 6am. I do get out in the community with other business owners, with friends, or kind of keep my personal connections that way, because once the day is over, I'm running around getting kids and all of that stuff. The morning is a really important time for me.

Please explain the most challenging time in your career and how you moved past it and thrived on the other side?

It was honestly when I got sued and had to go to small claim's court and represent myself. Now, in and of itself, I didn't do anything wrong and I got cleared. It was a joke. But that was challenging in the fact that not only did it bring extra stress into my life, but I was really more upset that you do everything you can for someone, you give it all you can, you are nice to them, bend over backwards, and do everything right clinically, and yet they're still not happy.

What we do is tough. We have to wear many hats. I think it really hardened me a little bit, I guess, as to the nature of humans, and doing the nice things and still getting sued for it. The other is that we did get embezzled by someone that I thought I could trust with my life.

Therefore, I've actually really pulled back even as a boss. I've put a wall up, to not get as personal with my team and trust them completely. That's probably bad, but on the other hand, you just never know. You hear about it time and time again.

How have I moved past it?

I feel like I haven't gotten hard, even with my team or my patients, but it has put me on guard. Where I'm at on the other side...I feel like we have awesome systems in place with the team, so that no one person is in charge, and I feel like it's allowed me to still provide for my patients, but kind of with a cautious air.

What is your goal-setting process?

My goal setting process is not really good. I know I'm supposed to be reading all of these business books. I know I'm supposed to be always working on myself professionally and personally, which I do. I just don't read a lot of books to do that. I probably should write down my goals. We do sit down every year and have something called the annual planning, in which we look at goals for how many days we're going to work, what our production goal is, and do we meet them? I'm constantly looking at numbers for patients, case acceptance. I think you need metrics. I want to get down to 3 days a week, and so I make it happen.

My personal mantra is, #makeithappen and #figureitout. I didn't write it down. I didn't set this goal by this date, but we now have an associate. We're sitting down next week to negotiate the contract. I feel like I just do it. I get a goal. I get my desire, and just make it happen.

There's probably a better system for that, but that's just kind of how I operate.

What is the best investment you have made either inside your career or outside of dentistry?

The best investment I made is going to dental school, and that's what you have to look at it as. It's not debt, but an investment; because otherwise, we wouldn't get to this point. However, the learning doesn't end there. I have not spent big numbers on CE, but I know that's an important component to your career.

I had young kids, and couldn't travel at the time, but I am making that investment now. I am going to sacrifice more of my time to make those CE courses. The best investment I made as an associate was paying for myself to go to the course in Dallas, TX with Kent Smith to learn sleep apnea.

My career would not be the same. To step out, to do something that no one else was doing around here so that I could learn to do it right. The other best investment I made is in home sleep tests. That's what has really grown that part of my business.

Also we recently purchased a CEREC and a CBCT. I would say—it may not have completely changed the way we practiced—however, it has made a difference. The 3D has definitely made a difference in the dentistry that we're doing and challenged us to elevate what we're providing for our patients, and not just run-of-the-mill fillings anymore.

Looking back, what advice would you give yourself on the day of your dental school graduation?

Find a mentor and find a mentor fast. Someone that you trust and respect. Someone that wants to be in that position. My dad was a dentist, and I was able to get some mentoring from him, but really, I could have dove in a whole lot more.

I would tell anybody graduating dental school to really check their ego at the door, and be open to learning, and be open to new ideas, and to not think that they have it all.

Especially the inter-personal relationship; the communication with patients, I think, is one thing that's hugely lacking. The other advice that I would give is to learn the business early. Learn it fast. Really learn how to lead your team, communicate with your team, and learn accounting and all of those things that we don't learn in dental school.

In your opinion, what separates the top 10% of dentists from the bottom 90%?

My opinion, what separates the top 10% of dentists from the bottom 90% is communication. Relationships. Being able to communicate what the patient needs, and being able to listen. Listen to what the patient wants, and tailor that treatment plan to them, or get them to see the value of what you're providing them. Bring them to that level of understanding.

Most patients, again, don't care about how much you know until they know how much you care.

What keeps struggling dentists struggling?

I really hope that I can articulate this correctly, because I have trained and helped a lot of dentists. The thing that gets in struggling dentists' way is the dentist. They drive me bonkers. They can't understand why they can't advance from where they're at, and that's because they overthink everything, question everything, and then don't move forward.

They don't change. The get so caught up in the weeds, that they don't see the big picture. I think that is just the culprit of many of our personalities, but I would say that dentists get in their own way.

Dave: *When I talk to dentists and they admit to feeling stuck, it generally is a byproduct of overthinking the next step and a clinging to the comfort zone. Peter Drucker says, "Marketing and innovation produce results; all the rest are costs." Marketing and practice innovation are two categories almost all of us can be stronger at.*

What are the top 3 books every dental practice owner should read?

I'm not big on business books. I did, however, read *Start with Why* [by Simon Sinek], and I think that is really important, because we need to know what to do and how to do it. We went to dental school, but we still need to create that culture of why. Getting the team onboard to see your vision, to create that environment that patients want to be a part of. I think that's the most important thing to growing your practice, and conveying that on social media, your websites, or in your community, is creating that why.

There is probably some other books that I should have read. One person that really did make a big difference in my communication is Ashley Latter. He wrote a book called *Don't Wait for the Tooth Fairy: How to Communicate*. He made a big difference in my career as well.

If you had to narrow it down to a couple...what traits or skills do you think are most important in running an uncommonly successful practice?

Communication and listening. Simple as that.

What is a skill or procedure you've added since graduating from dental school that has had a major positive impact on your practice?

Obviously, sleep apnea. Huge impact! Changed my life, and changes other people's lives. It's truly a huge passion of mine that they don't teach you in dental school.

What is the best business advice you ever received?

Find and surround yourself with the experts. You don't have to be the expert at everything, but surround yourself by those that can either give you advice, or just do the work for you, so you don't have to be good at everything.

What advice would you give a dentist that is struggling with case acceptance?

I think that many times the dentist talks too much. There is a reason that God gave us 1 mouth and 2 ears. Ethical Sales and Communication with Ashley Latter, is what really kind of spelled it out for me.

Emotionally connect that patient to their oral health, to their mouth, to their smile, to their sleep. Emotional connection, listening to their story, and bringing them to a point where they value what you're providing them, and finding the treatment plan that works best for them, and not just thinking that the objection is always money.

I think we compromise treatment plans, thinking that the patient would never go for it. I think we compromise treatment plans, thinking that the patient wouldn't want to go through all of that effort. Find out what the objection is, and overcome it. I would say that my case acceptance has gone through the roof because of that.

It's listening to the patient, and kind of bringing that conversation to that specific patient, tailoring it to them, so that you can get the treatment plan that means both walk away with a win-win.

What marketing advice would you give a dentist that is starting out in practice ownership?

The marketing advice I would give is not to just throw everything at the wall and see what sticks. Obviously, it's knowing your demographic. Who is your target audience? Once you establish that, what is the best way to reach them?

Whatever your target demographic is, once you identify that, find the in-roads. The social media that we do really portrays our culture, so that patients want to be a part of it.

If they like a homey, fun, family-friendly environment, that's us. If they want a high society, sterile environment, then we're not for them. Conveying who you are to the public is really my advice for you.

Dave: I think too many dental marketing companies deliver a one-size fits all product. People are attracted by personality in marketing...or they may be repelled (but you wouldn't want that patient anyway; it's not a match to your practice culture).

What do our dental patients most desire?

I think patients most desire to be cared about and know that you are good at what you do, but you care about them.

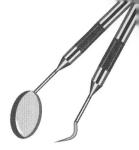

DR. TARUN AGARWAL

Raleigh Dental Arts, 3D Dentists

Justin: I've listened to Tarun speak many times and have always liked that he calls it the way he sees it!

Background

Dr. Tarun Agarwal is a respected speaker, author, and opinion leader; he is changing the way general dentists practice. His common-sense approach to business, dedication to clinical excellence, integration of technology, and down-to-earth demeanor has made him a recognized educator.

Scratch Private Practice 2001
Co-Founder Townie Meeting 2002
Founder 3D Dentists 2013

Please explain your style of practice (practice size, location, procedure mix, etc.)

Raleigh, NC—general practice providing nearly all services to patients. We are 2 dentists and 9 team members. My main focus is complex restorative dentistry, implant dentistry, and sleep apnea therapy. My associate dentist does the majority of general dentistry and ortho-dontic services.

Do you have a favorite success quote or mantra?

If you're not moving forward, you're moving backwards.

In regards to your dental career, what would you like your legacy to be, or how would you like to be remembered?

That I empowered general dentists to build the practice they dreamed they would have in dental school.

What does success mean to you?

Making an impact on those around me to achieve their life goals. This includes my team members, other dentists, and my family.

What is your morning routine (first 1–2 hrs of the day)?

I spend the first 30 minutes in random thoughts. Then I spend 45 minutes in light exercise/activity.

What is your biggest fear?

Failure.

Please explain the most challenging time in your career and how you moved past it and thrived on the other side?

When I nearly went bankrupt trying to build a fee-for-service cash practice. I stopped listening to "gurus" and trying to be something I wasn't. I started taking insurance, but never lost sight of the long-term goal. In other words, I didn't let insurance dictate how we treated people.

Justin: *I think this is a great lesson for everyone to take note of. Sometimes you have to follow your gut and make the necessary pivots to reach the level of success you want to achieve.*

What is your goal-setting process?

Most people set their annual goals in January. I believe that is too late. I start my goal setting in August. This allows me to reflect on the current year, set goals based on reality, and put things in place to achieve the goals for the following year. I set the conceptual goal and then work backwards on what it takes to make it happen. You must be very specific and realistic.

What is the best investment you have made either inside your career or outside of dentistry?

My parents gave me $10k for graduation with the caveat that I must use it on education. I took so much CE my first year out of school, and it has paid off like I couldn't have imagined.

Justin: I plan on stealing this idea for my children. What a great idea and gift!

Looking back, what advice would you give yourself on the day of your dental school graduation?

You have enough education to sustain you for 6 months. Just continue to learn and expand your clinical skill set.

In your opinion, what separates the top 10% of dentists from the bottom 90%?

Communication. The logical and typical answer is leadership, but leadership is just communication.

What keeps struggling dentists struggling?

Lack of passion in their profession.

What are the top 3 books every dental practice owner should read?

Making it Easy for Patients to Say "Yes" by Paul Homoly
Good to Great by Jim Collins
Expert Secrets by Russel Brunson

If you had to narrow it down to a couple...what traits or skills do you think are most important in running an uncommonly successful practice?

Communication. Being different. Quick to fire the wrong hires.

What is a skill or procedure you've added since graduating from dental school that has had a major positive impact on your practice?

Dental implants.

What is the best business advice you ever received?

You can't save your way to riches. You have to produce your way to it. My father told me that you can only reduce costs but so much; the real key is to figure out how to expand your revenue.

Dave: *Agreed. There have been a few times in my career that I got overly focused on cutting overhead. Playing defense was pretty ineffective for me. It triggered a scarcity mindset and had negative effects on my top line...which of course, negatively affected my bottom line. I'm happier and more prosperous when I focus my efforts completely on practice growth!*

What leadership advice would you give a dentist who has an ineffective culture in their practice?

They must first design their ideal practice and write it down. Then start living that culture and make the tough decisions to let those around you who don't live that culture go.

What advice would you give a dentist that is struggling with case acceptance?

Learn to earn the trust of patients. Become a patient advocate.

What marketing advice would you give a dentist that is starting out in practice ownership?

Leverage dental insurance and don't market general dentistry. Market those services that most dentists aren't doing.

What do our dental patients most desire?

A trusting place.

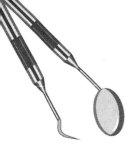

DR. BILL BLATCHFORD

Blatchford Solutions

Justin: *Where do I begin with this introduction? Bill is one of the top 2 mentors in my career. Bill was my first coach in dentistry and pushed me to break through the multitude of glass ceilings I had in my career and life. I owe a lot to Bill.*

Bill also gave me the first taste of being able to coach others many years ago, which at this point has become a big part of my life. We've talked and stayed in touch after almost 12 years, and I can't say enough good things about him. I know he doesn't do these kinds of things often, but I'm honored that he agreed to be a part of this book!

Background

I grew up on a dairy farm in Western Oregon. Always interested in science; and a love of animals led me to study pre-vet at Washington State University. While there, I spent time with dentists who shared their enthusiasm for dentistry. It was life changing. I graduated from Loyola Dental School in Chicago. I started a private practice in Corvallis, Oregon in 1970. I loved practicing dentistry. I was able to grow the practice to over $1,000,000 by the mid-80s. I found that taking care of the patients and team from a service mentality was equally as important as the clinical side. With the help of several consultants, we were able to develop systems to make the practice efficient and profitable.

I found that other dentists wanted to learn what I was doing. I was a CE junkie, so I constantly met dentists from all over the country that wanted help. I invited them to the office to observe what I was doing. I enjoyed this.

In 1990, after much discussion with my wife Carolyn, we decided to sell the practice and start our own consulting business. I started by setting up small groups of dentists in several Western Canada and US cities. I would fly my plane to each city every month to meet with them. We also did seminars, and I actually visited all the offices. Over the years, I have spoken at most of the major meetings in the US and Canada. I have been fortunate to have also traveled to speak in many foreign countries.

Our business has grown over the years to its present model. Two years ago, we sold the business to our daughter, Dr. Christina Blatchford. I still enjoy the interaction with the clients. My wife still enjoys writing articles and books. We have published 5 books on practice management. Our younger daughter also works in the business, doing logistics for meetings and marketing.

Currently we are enjoying our 3 grandchildren. Carolyn and I have been married 50 years and are looking forward to 30 more years on this planet. We enjoy traveling, skiing, and spending 2 months on our boat in the Northwest and Canadian coast to Alaska. We also spend 2 months at our home in Mexico.

Please explain your style of practice (practice size, location, procedure mix, etc.)

I have developed several really efficient systems for dental practices and emphasize the leadership skills of the doctor. Our clients are able to have balance in their lives because they spend less time in the office than most. They also earn a better income while providing their patients with excellent care.

Do you have a favorite success quote or mantra?

Life is a banquet; lick your platter clean.

In regards to your dental career, what would you like your legacy to be, or how would you like to be remembered?

Balance of all areas of one's life.

What does success mean to you?

Ability to pursue one's dreams, whatever they are.

What is your morning routine (first 1–2 hrs of the day)?

Exercise at the nearby health club. Carolyn and I do this together. Eat breakfast together and discuss the objectives of the day. We also express our gratitude for this great life.

What is your biggest fear?

I really do not have any.

Please explain the most challenging time in your career and how you moved past it and thrived on the other side?

Just after 9/11, our business really suffered because it was seminar based and required clients to travel to us. No one wanted to get on an airplane. Lots of refunds as team members would not travel. We call it the great potato famine. We just worked our way through this difficult time. I also had a very loyal team who believed in our message and us. I could not have done this without the support of our family and team.

What is your goal-setting process?

We have always set long-term goals first. We have quantified the goals. What is enjoyable at this stage is that we have met most of the goals we have set and are continually setting new goals for our life.

What is the best investment you have made either inside your career or outside of dentistry?

The time spent with our family.

Looking back, what advice would you give yourself on the day of your dental school graduation?

Live within your means and pay off all debt.

In your opinion, what separates the top 10% of dentists from the bottom 90%?

Attitude.

What keeps struggling dentists struggling?

They are committed to struggle. The glass is half empty.

What are the top 3 books every dental practice owner should read?

The 7 Habits of Successful People by Covey.

Dave: *I like that Bill just answered with one. Seven Habits is also my #1. It changed my life radically when I was an undergrad.*

If you had to narrow it down to a couple...what traits or skills do you think are most important in running an uncommonly successful practice?

Leadership, which is a learned skill.

What is the best business advice you ever received?

Life first. Practice to support it.

Dave: *So many of our colleagues get this backwards. We've talked on the RD podcast from day one that an epic practice needs to serve your epic life, however you choose to define that.*

What leadership advice would you give a dentist who has an ineffective culture in their practice?

Write a vision statement and live it.

What advice would you give a dentist that is struggling with case acceptance?

Take our program and study sales.

What marketing advice would you give a dentist that is starting out in practice ownership?

Everything you do is marketing. Make sure the message is correct.

Dave: Everything is Marketing *by Fred Joyal is a book that I've given all new hires in my practice. I want them to understand that there is no neutral when it comes to patient perception. Everything we do is judged as a plus or a minus. I should also mention that I leaned heavily on Bill's books when starting my practice in 2009–10. They're filled with unique practice strategies that I haven't heard any other dental thought leaders discuss.*

What do our dental patients most desire?

Look good, feel good, and value.

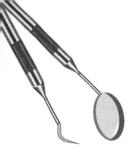

DR. JUSTIN MOODY

The Dental Implant Center, Implant Pathway, Podcaster

Dave: *I admire Justin for many reasons. He's funny, generous, and a talented clinician and educator. He's synergized teaching dentists implants while giving a helping hand to veterans and the homeless. Plus, he's a fellow podcaster and a fellow Nebraska Farm Boy. Go Big Red!*

Background

Dr. Justin Moody is the fifth generation to be raised on the Moody family ranch in Northwest Nebraska. He attended the University of Nebraska and received his doctorate at the University of Oklahoma College of Dentistry. He returned to his hometown of Crawford, Nebraska upon graduation in 1997, where he opened his first practice; today he owns and operates 6 offices in 2 states.

Since graduation, Dr. Moody has been active in continuing education and implant dentistry, and in 2008, he limited his practice to the field of dental implants. He is a Diplomate of the American Board of Oral Implantology, a Diplomate, Master, and Fellow with the International Congress of Oral Implantology; Fellow and Associate Fellow with the American Academy of Implant Dentistry; Adjunct Professor at the

University of Nebraska Medical Center; Kois Center Mentor; and a member of the Dentistry Today Implant Advisory Board.

Dr. Moody is in private practice; his company Implant Pathway provides dental education across the country; and he is active in the dental podcast world where you can catch him on his show called *Dentists, Implants, and Worms*—as well as the *AAID Podcast*. His real passion is for helping those less fortunate receive dental care while mentoring dentists to be better; he recently founded the New Horizons Institute in Phoenix, Arizona to do just that.

Please explain your style of practice (practice size, location, procedure mix, etc.)

My practice is limited to dental implants; in 2008, I moved from my hometown of Crawford, Nebraska to Rapid City, South Dakota to open The Dental Implant Center. What is unique about this is that it's a referral-based business; we have about 45 doctors in 4 states that send us their dental implant patients. I have 5 other general dentistry offices that my management team oversees and runs, while I provide the mentorship and advanced implant treatment.

Do you have a favorite success quote or mantra?

"Today I will do what others won't,
so tomorrow I can accomplish what others can't."

—JERRY RICE

In regards to your dental career, what would you like your legacy to be, or how would you like to be remembered?

My hope is that when I finish my career, I have made a difference in at least one dentist's life. That difference could translate to hundreds if not thousands of patients receiving better care and services; that's a legacy.

What does success mean to you?

Success is not measured in dollars or cars to me; it's in the number of friends you meet and the relationships you build.

Dave: *I've been honored to speak at a couple of conferences with Justin. In those presentations, I recall him saying that the knowledge you take from a CE event is important, but leaving with more friends than you came with is even more valuable. A powerful message I took to heart.*

What is your morning routine (first 1–2 hrs of the day)?

I am at the office at 5:45am every morning; it's my 2 hours of alone time. I spend 30 minutes reading journals or online articles, the next 60 minutes answering emails and study club questions, and the balance of the time in social media connecting, networking, and posting.

What is your biggest fear?

Only things that are not in my control.

Please explain the most challenging time in your career and how you moved past it and thrived on the other side?

April 14th, 2014 to be exact. In 2011, I had a vision of opening a dental implant training center in downtown Denver, Colorado; this vision turned into reality in 2012 and was called the Rocky Mountain Dental Institute.

It was my "field of dreams"; however, not enough people came. Was plagued with hiring the wrong personnel, a tough economic time, and the fact that no one had really heard of me yet, a cart before the horse deal. At the same time the teaching center was failing, so were many of my practices, due to a lack of leadership, since I was always gone. That time in my life was filled with potential bankruptcy attorneys, consultants—it was just one large dumpster fire. April 14th was the day I packed up the teaching center and left the dream in downtown Denver.

What is your goal-setting process?

Goals are not my thing, as they seem so finite; seems like every time I am about to reach one, the project turns another direction. I am more about vision than goals.

What is the best investment you have made either inside your career or outside of dentistry?

Education; learning from everyone is key. None of us are smarter than all of us.

Looking back, what advice would you give yourself on the day of your dental school graduation?

Never stop learning, never stop meeting people, never stop dreaming.

In your opinion, what separates the top 10% of dentists from the bottom 90%?

Communication skills; if you think about it, the patient doesn't really know good work from bad. If the dentist can communicate the issues in a way that shows the patient the need and value of their services, then most patients will figure out how to do it. It's that simple.

What keeps struggling dentists struggling?

Arrogance and ego.

What are the top 3 books every dental practice owner should read?

The Tipping Point by Malcolm Gladwell
Start with Why by Simon Sinek
The Pumpkin Plan by Mike Michalowicz

If you had to narrow it down to a couple...what traits or skills do you think are most important in running an uncommonly successful practice?

Communication skills and the ability to recognize areas that you are weak in, so you can ask for help.

What is a skill or procedure you've added since graduating from dental school that has had a major positive impact on your practice?

Dental implants, hands down. It is the only true tooth-replacement solution we have in dentistry today. The ability to give someone back their smile, ability to eat, and the confidence to not have their floating dentures fly out of their mouth is life changing to the patient and career satisfying to me.

What is the best business advice you ever received?

You are your own self limiter; if you want to do something in life, only you can stop that dream. I have carried that through to all of my projects in life and have no regrets about where I am.

What leadership advice would you give a dentist who has an ineffective culture in their practice?

Remove the cancer; it's always someone that doesn't see your vision or share in your values that simmers under the surface, keeping everyone from enjoying the workplace. You have to practice what you preach, first one to work, last one to leave, and never delegate something you are not willing to do yourself.

What advice would you give a dentist that is struggling with case acceptance?

Education and communication training. I know I sound like a broken record, but the only way to have good case acceptance is to have good communication skills.

What marketing advice would you give a dentist that is starting out in practice ownership?

Surround yourself with people you trust and people who fill in the gaps where you are not the expert. Problem is you may not know these areas yet; just keep an open mind and ask for help when you need it.

What do our dental patients most desire?

To be treated well, and to know that we care.

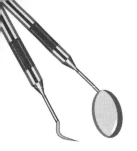

DR. HOWARD FARRAN

Today's Dental; founder of Dentaltown

Justin: *Dentaltown has become an icon in the dental world, just like its founder, Howard Farran. In true Howard fashion, he keeps it real, and I think there is a lot of wisdom in his words on finding and empowering the right people. I got to wake Howard up early on a Sunday morning to do this interview, but he was very gracious and it was great getting to connect with him.*

Dave: *I first learned about the business of dentistry from Howard and his 30-Day Dental MBA series. My good friend, Dr. Ryan Foote, had shipped me a huge box of VHS tapes to my house in Germany in 2003. I remember watching those tapes with fascination. I thank Howard for laying down that foundation of strong business systems and practice management long before I would actually start my own practice in 2009.*

Background

In 1998, I was on the internet, watching people talk about football in the ESPN forums, and I thought, "Damn, man—we should be talking about root canals, fillings, and crowns." So the next day, I hired Ken Scott to program, and that was the genesis of Dentaltown.

Since then, we have never signed up less than 1,000 dentists a month. Now DT has more than 250,000 users from 200 countries. It began as me just wanting to talk to another dentist.

Please explain your style of practice (practice size, location, procedure mix, etc.)

I started practicing in Phoenix in 1987; I consider my specialty to be public health. I tell my patients that if they have a problem, they can come on down and I'll fix it. That's where I came up with the name for my practice: Today's Dental. Just like a fireman won't tell someone, "Sorry, I can't put out your fire because I'm getting ready to go to lunch,"—I have an op that we don't schedule that's open for unscheduled treatments, and that's always been my secret sauce.

Do you have a favorite success quote or mantra?

It doesn't make sense to hire the best people in the world and then micromanage them. Hire the best people you can find, and then get out of their way.

In regard to your dental career, what would you like your legacy to be, or how would you like to be remembered?

I'd like to be remembered in my practice as a fireman or a policeman. If my patients have a "dental fire" that needs to be put out 20 minutes before closing, I'm going to stay and put out that fire and take care of them. There is a lot of entitlement in dentistry these days; dentists want to work only cookie-cutter hours, and public health is not a cookie-cutter field.

What does "success" mean to you?

If you asked me if I was successful, I'd say I'm completely successful, because I've never worked a day in my life.

I grew up so poor that I didn't even know some people had air conditioners. I started working in my dad's Sonic drive-in at 10 years old. I didn't want to go home and sit around the house, so I thought I was the luckiest kid around. I learned everything about business from working with my dad. I think that free enterprise, business, treating your customer better, and trying to figure out how you can give them something faster, easier, lower cost, and higher quality is the most exciting thing in the world and I love every minute of it.

What is your morning routine (first 1–2 hours of the day)?

I get up and check my emails; I get around 300 a day. I love getting emails from dentists all over the world and giving them access to free continuing education on Dentaltown. The ability to transfer the knowledge from the oldest, richest dentists in America to a poor dentist in Ethiopia is amazing.

What is your biggest fear?

Living in fear is not an option. We're all going to die, so living in fear has never been an option. When I started Dentaltown and people told me we couldn't compete with the established publications, I told them we couldn't live in fear, and we went out and did it.

What is your goal-setting process?

It has changed. Thirty years ago when I started my practice, it was about me; now, it's about figuring out what my team needs. My business is my family, and I try to figure out what they need.

What is the best investment you have made, either inside your career or outside of dentistry?

Investing in myself. Why would you want to put all your money in some stock that could implode? The bottom line is, you only have one life—why don't you invest all the money in yourself? If you're really passionate about sleep apnea, chairside milling, or lasers, invest in yourself and be all you can be. Why invest your money in a company that has an 88% mortality rate over 65 years? YOU should be the greatest company in the world.

Looking back, what advice would you give yourself on the day of your dental school graduation?

Find the best damn people, and keep and retain them. If you have the best damn people, you'll build the best damn business!

In your opinion, what separates the top 10% of dentists from the bottom 90%?

Doing what you're passionate about. You should be willing to do whatever you're doing for free, if you had to. Don't do things you don't like to do for money. Ask yourself why you wanted to be a dentist and find that passion—that is your secret sauce!

What keeps struggling dentists struggling?

Imagine you own a restaurant, and you're the chef of all chefs, and you keep wanting to add new items and recipes. Then imagine there is another chef who says, "To hell with it—people are going to come in for the pizza, beef stroganoff, or whatever. I only need a few hot items and I'm going to crush it with the employees."

Your clientele all comes back for the consistency. They know they're going to get a good meal, and see the same maître d', the same waitress, etc.

I would bet all my money on the person who masters the people skills, not the dental skills.

If you had to narrow it down to a couple, what traits or skills do you think are most important in running an uncommonly successful practice?

Being a human. Instead of being that dentist who finishes that procedure and then goes back to their office and shuts the door, stay out there and bond with that patient, or your team members. You have to be able to sell the invisible—it's the dentists who have the best chairside personality, or who personally apologize to a patient for running behind, who are going to be fine. If you can have sympathy and empathy and you're connected to your staff and your patients, you're going to crush it.

What is a skill or procedure you've added since graduating from dental school that has had a major positive impact on your practice?

Root canals. All these people say they want to add sleep apnea, bone grafts, implants, but all that is bullshit. People come in with a toothache and they need a root canal, but so many dentists just refer that to an endodontist. It's just insanity. You're a dentist, they have a toothache, they need a root canal. Learn how to do root canals!

Dave: *LOL. Howard pulls no punches.*

What is the best business advice you ever received?

Attract and retain people who understand people, time, and money, and then get out of their way.

What advice would you give a dentist who is struggling with case acceptance?

When you watch a football game, and there are 50 employees and coaches on each side, they each give their best, and at the end of the game, someone still loses. There has to be a score. Only one-third of cavities get drilled, filled, and billed. If you have someone on your team that can get two-thirds, empower them and get out of their way.

What do our dental patients most desire?

Half of our patients are afraid of dentistry, and the other half are afraid of the dental bill. You need to be able to put patients at ease, and give patients options so they can afford the dentistry.

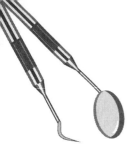

DR. JOHN NOSTI

Smile Design NYC,
Clinical Mastery

Background

Dr. John Nosti graduated from Stockton University prior to attending Rutgers School of Dental Medicine. He then went on to complete a one-year GPR at Lehigh Valley Hospital in Allentown, PA. He has since amassed well over 2000 hours of CE in 20 years of practice.

He has earned fellowships from the Academy of General Dentistry, Academy of Comprehensive Esthetics, and International Congress of Oral Implantologists. Dr. Nosti is currently the Clinical Director for the Clinical Mastery Series, a continuum dedicated to advancing the confidence and competency of dentists worldwide in cosmetic and rehabilitation dentistry. In short, we teach others how to #RockTheDrill. He has been consistently named a "top speaker" in Continuing Education, as well as a "Top Dentist" in New Jersey, where he practices full time.

He is married to his wife Jen and has 2 children, a daughter Isabella, and a son AJ (Anthony Joseph). As a lifelong commitment to health, Dr. Nosti is a certified personal trainer and weight management specialist. He and his wife Jen opened their first "Anytime Fitness" center in the fall of 2017.

In his free time, John loves to spend time with his family.

Please explain your style of practice (practice size, location, procedure mix, etc.)

I have 2 locations that I share with a partner. We have a general dental practice with a focus on cosmetic and rehabilitation dentistry.

Do you have a favorite success quote or mantra?

Victory is reserved for those who are willing to pay the price.

In regards to your dental career, what would you like your legacy to be, or how would you like to be remembered?

From my patients—I would love them to remember me as someone who cared for them, made their visits easier, and as someone who gave them the confidence to smile. From fellow dentists—I would love them to remember me as someone who made practicing complex dentistry easier and a lot more fun!

Justin: I first met John at a Clinical Mastery course that he was an instructor at. I can say that he made my complex cases easier, and he is a wonderful down-to-earth instructor!

What does success mean to you?

Love what you do! Be able to practice the way you want to practice, performing the type of dentistry you want to perform, which allows you endless opportunities in your personal life. Spending time with the family!

What is your morning routine (first 1–2 hrs of the day)?

Working out! It helps me set up my energy for the day by starting me out on a positive note.

What is your biggest fear?

Heights...haha.

Please explain the most challenging time in your career and how you moved past it and thrived on the other side?

I think one of the biggest challenges we face is seeing our own dentistry fail. I can tell you regardless of what the cause was/is, I have a tendency to take this personally and feel that it is somehow my fault. I believe this comes from an expectation put on us in dental school that your dentistry should last forever. Learning that everything has a life expectancy, and patients play an enormous role in the success outcomes, was one of the most challenging things for me to learn.

What is your goal-setting process?

I think it is important to routinely set goals for yourself professionally and personally. When I do decide on a short-term or long-term goal, I commit it to paper and review it routinely until it is achieved! I feel the consistent reviewing and reminding yourself of your goals is something that will help you conquer them.

What is the best investment you have made either inside your career or outside of dentistry?

In quality continuing education. In short, I invested in myself!

Looking back, what advice would you give yourself on the day of your dental school graduation?

I like the path that I took: dedicate yourself to quality CE, set goals, and continue to grow. Outside of dentistry—buy stock in Amazon and Google.

In your opinion, what separates the top 10% of dentists from the bottom 90%?

Confidence.

Justin: *Confidence is a recurring theme in response to this question.*

What keeps struggling dentists struggling?

I feel it is lack of goals, leadership, and confidence. There are ways to build a top-performing office anywhere...seek the advice of others and don't reinvent the wheel.

What are the top 3 books every dental practice owner should read?

Change Your Questions, Change Your Life by Marilee Adams
How to Win Friends and Influence People by Dale Carnegie
Success Principles by Jack Canfield

If you had to narrow it down to a couple...what traits or skills do you think are most important in running an uncommonly successful practice?

I feel it is important to be friendly/honest, patient, a good communicator, and be a good leader to your team. I think these three traits come above one's skills. You can be a great clinician, but without having these three traits I think you won't do as well as the person who does.

What is a skill or procedure you've added since graduating from dental school that has had a major positive impact on your practice?

Having patience and being a good communicator. Being able to sit knee to knee, eye to eye and have a conversation with someone who genuinely feels you have their best interests in mind is what I feels separates me from many other doctors out there.

Having patience, not letting your emotions get the better of you, and staying calm while communicating is a skill everyone needs to learn.

What is the best business advice you ever received?

The best advice, invest in yourself. Second, would be to make sure you have a low overhead.

What leadership advice would you give a dentist who has an ineffective culture in their practice?

Don't tolerate poor attitude on your team! The situation will only get worse over time and good employees will become ineffective to match the poor-performing staff members. Staph (staff) is an infection that you don't want—TEAM is what you want. Have meetings and set the expectations of each employee. Those who don't meet your expectations are shown the door.

Dave: *In my experience, something amazing happens when someone with a poor attitude is shown the door. The rest of the team gets better immediately. You assume that you'll be short-handed but the rest of the team steps up, fills in gaps, and often out-produces the larger team.*

What advice would you give a dentist that is struggling with case acceptance?

First—you have to be well educated in comprehensive dentistry. I feel that having a solid education will allow you to present treatment plans confidently. When you question yourself in your mind, patients will question your abilities.

Once you have a sound education and believe in the dentistry you provide, the next step is to read the book *Change your Questions,*

Change your Life. It isn't always about how well you answer your patient's questions; it is sometimes the great questions you ask them. We are taught we always need to have an answer, and when it comes to case acceptance, that just isn't always the case.

Justin: *Great book, and I would agree the ability to ask the right questions had a profound effect on my case acceptance during my career.*

What marketing advice would you give a dentist that is starting out in practice ownership?

Have a good quality website, so you are visible online. I truly feel it is important to build from the inside with word of mouth. Make sure you are friendly and approachable, and spend time talking with people and explaining things to them in a manner they understand. When patients compliment you or your staff, ask them to refer their friends and family to your office. The website is so that people can do their homework and check you out when others have referred them to you.

What do our dental patients most desire?

Being treated kindly. I think most patients to this day still hate the dentist. Make their appointment enjoyable, and you will succeed.

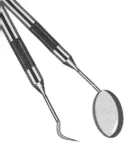

DR. LEE ANN BRADY

Desert Sun Smiles,
The Pankey Institute

Justin: *At the end of each of these interviews, we asked each doctor to mention someone we should make sure is included in this book. Lee's name kept reappearing, which speaks volumes.*

Although I hadn't met Dr. Brady in person, I have known of her for quite some time. She was another one where I just naively assumed her dental career was all up and to the right. I was surprised to learn she had quit dentistry for a few years, and I'm grateful she was open enough to tell her story. I know she is not the only one that has felt the way she has in the past, and it's inspiring to hear how she persevered through and regained her love of dentistry.

Background

Dr. Lee Ann Brady earned her D.M.D. degree from the University of Florida, College of Dentistry. Dr. Brady was invited to join the Pankey Institute as their first female resident faculty member and was promoted to Clinical Director within a year. She held the position of Clinical Director until November of 2008 and is currently a guest faculty presenter at The Pankey Institute.

She was asked by Dr. Frank Spear to join him in the formation of Spear Education and the expansion of his curriculum in the fall of 2008. As the Executive VP of Clinical Education at Spear Education until June of 2011, she managed the development and delivery of all programs.

After leaving Spear Education, she launched LeeAnnBrady.com, which provides daily clinical and practice management articles and short videos. Dr. Brady served as the Director of Education for the Clinical Mastery series from 2014–2017. RestorativeNation.com, an online learning community, was launched in February of 2017, featuring video content, live webinars, and online community support through forum discussion.

In May of 2017, she rejoined The Pankey Institute as Director of Education. Dr. Brady owns Desert Sum Smiles, a private restorative practice in Glendale, AZ where she sees patients 10–12 days per month. She has served on the editorial review boards of the Seattle Study Club Journal, Inside Dentistry, DentalTown Magazine, and The Journal of Cosmetic Dentistry. Dr. Brady has been published in numerous journals.

Please explain your style of practice (practice size, location, procedure mix, etc.)

Private restorative practice, serving primarily adult patients. We have about 1000 active patients, 25% TMD, 30% Advanced Restorative, and 45% more general prosth and operative procedures.

Do you have a favorite success quote or mantra?

Not really. I never set out to achieve most of the things I have. I simply put one foot in front of the other everyday, handled the tasks in front of me, and considered the opportunities ahead of me. Somehow, you look back after 30 years and go, wow, I did all of that.

In regards to your dental career, what would you like your legacy to be, or how would you like to be remembered?

If I can help other dentists to figure out how to love our profession and gain all the success and fulfillment from it that they seek. Dentistry can be tough, technically and psychologically, and yet to the outside world, people miss that part. We do have the gift of being able to customize our experience, yet most of us don't take advantage of this freedom.

What does success mean to you?

Success is not one thing or simple. I have figured out how to love my career and how to be good at it, so I can serve my patients and all the dentists I get to teach.

The success piece is the journey, working hard and sticking with it for me, not the outcome. I also have a fantastic husband and 3 incredible young adults that I had the pleasure to raise. Again for me, success is the stories and the shared journey I have traveled with my family and includes both the ups and the downs. I guess in the end, success is walking my own path and creating my own story.

What is your morning routine (first 1–2 hrs of the day)?

I get up early; it's an old habit that gave me time by myself before my family was awake and I had to deal with work. I make myself a cup of coffee and have "me" time for awhile. Then I get ready to face the day.

What is your biggest fear?

Not being relevant.

Please explain the most challenging time in your career and how you moved past it and thrived on the other side?

I left dentistry in 1999. I had practiced in several different ways, including my own private practice and truly hated it. I felt trapped everyday when I went to work. The technical dentistry wasn't working, the practice was always a challenge, and I wasn't happy. I thought there was no way to enjoy dentistry, so I sold my practice and was out of the profession for 2.5 years.

I went back to work as a dentist as an associate when my husband lost his job. I landed in the practice of a dentist who had a very different approach, and I figured out very quickly that I was loving practicing this way. This was the beginning of my incredible relationship with continuing education, first as a student and then as an instructor.

What is your goal-setting process?

I schedule quiet time—sometimes it is a whole day—where my husband and I can get away, and we simply daydream, and brainstorm about the future. It is a loose structure, but it holds the boundaries of the direction we are headed. We have done this together for many years.

What is the best investment you have made either inside your career or outside of dentistry?

Significant continuing education.

Looking back, what advice would you give yourself on the day of your dental school graduation?

Always be a student, stay engaged, learn, and always be curious about what is possible.

In your opinion, what separates the top 10% of dentists from the bottom 90%?

Engagement in our profession beyond the walls of their offices, being in relationship with other dentists, and always striving to better themselves and our profession.

What keeps struggling dentists struggling?

Isolation; dentistry is a tough profession and only another dentist can understand and help. If we get into our offices and try to do the same things over and over, hoping they will become more predictable, then we struggle both technically and psychologically.

Dave: *Technology gives us so many mediums in which we can communicate and collaborate. Dentists who feel alone, stuck, and isolated can now easily find peer groups that will support one another without having to leave home.*

What are the top 3 books every dental practice owner should read?

The Art of Possibility by Rosamund Zander
The Energy of Money by Maria Nemeth
A Philosophy of the Practice of Dentistry by Pankey and Davis

If you had to narrow it down to a couple...what traits or skills do you think are most important in running an uncommonly successful practice?

Listening, self-understanding, and patience.

What is a skill or procedure you've added since graduating from dental school that has had a major positive impact on your practice?

TMD/Occlusal Therapy

What is the best business advice you ever received?

Learn to understand and run a business; it's a skill, but you need to be trained.

What leadership advice would you give a dentist who has an ineffective culture in their practice?

First work on yourself, figure out what you want, then learn to help others want that with you.

Dave: *Leading ourselves is most difficult. But, I agree with Dr. Brady, it's the right place to start!*

What advice would you give a dentist that is struggling with case acceptance?

Listening is the most important skill in case acceptance. Get to know your patients.

What marketing advice would you give a dentist that is starting out in practice ownership?

Strong patient relationships are key. Do what you do very well so people want you to be their provider.

What do our dental patients most desire?

It's not one thing; different people want different things, but knowing that is the key.

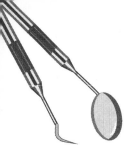

DR. DEREK WILLIAMS

The Lifestyle Practice,
Lufkin Family Dental

Justin: *I know Derek pretty well as he's recently become my partner at The Lifestyle Practice. Derek is one of those outliers that was probably born a go-getter. I think he was more prepared for practice ownership at graduation than I was 5 years into private practice. He was able to retire his $300K in school debt his first year out of school. It has been a joy to see him grow his practice and accomplish so much in a short amount of time. He has become a great asset for younger doctors looking to get into practice ownership and grow their practice and life at a fast clip.*

Background

I've always been an entrepreneur at heart. At 12 years old, I created flyers, with great incentives, to sign up for a season of lawn-mowing with me and delivered them across my neighborhood.

After reading, *Rich Dad Poor Dad* in high school, I became determined to learn how to make my money work for me. I wanted to have a life driven by passion and fulfillment, not tied down to a job.

My ultimate achievement has been my family. I'm married and have 4 daughters. They are my ultimate source of joy. My motivation to become financially independent is fueled by my desire to spend more time with them.

Please explain your style of practice (practice size, location, procedure mix, etc.)

I purchased a practice right out of dental school. I am located in East Texas. My practice has 4 operatories; I work out of 2 and have 2 hygienists. Procedures I perform include: fillings, crown and bridge, RCT, implants, clear correct, dentures. I do the simple cases and refer out the more difficult ones.

Do you have a favorite success quote or mantra?

Work hard, Play hard.

In regards to your dental career, what would you like your legacy to be, or how would you like to be remembered?

I would like to be remembered by my patients as being willing to take the time to explain Tx, allowing patients to make their own decisions. Helping patients to maintain their dentition by prevention.

What does success mean to you?

Working to achieve your goals.

What is your morning routine (first 1–2 hrs of the day)?

My normal routine is that I get woken up by my kids, get ready, eat breakfast and read scriptures with my kids, take my daughter to school, and head to work.

What is your biggest fear?

Not reaching my potential. I struggle with finding a balance between being happy with my achievements and the fear that I could have done better.

Please explain the most challenging time in your career and how you moved past it and thrived on the other side?

The first few months in practice ownership (and as a dentist) were very challenging. I lost about 25 lbs because I woke up with my stomach turning every day. I remember talking to Justin Short (my coach) about how overwhelming everything was: clinical, staff management, managing overhead, etc.

He told me that if I stayed the course, this would soon pass, and I would soon get to the point where I didn't think about work much outside of being at work. Here I am one year later, and that prophecy has been fulfilled. I've been able to pay off all school debt, my practice has doubled inside of 12 months, and I've been able to go from working 4 days a week to 3. I enjoy my time at home and am able to live in the moment with my wife and kids.

Justin: I can confirm this story. I still remember that phone call with Derek. Derek was featured on 2 podcasts with Shared Practices. One was in his first month as an owner, and one a year later. If you listen to those, the transformation you hear in his voice alone is pretty awesome. You can tell how he had grown as a practice owner. On Derek's behalf, I will say the changes in his practice, and the growth he experienced, did not happen by chance. The guy put in the work, and it's paid off, and he's reaping the rewards, already, in his career.

What is your goal-setting process?

I enjoy having 3 different timeframe categories for goals. They should all coincide with each other. I have daily and monthly goals, yearly goals, and long-term goals. My daily and monthly goals are set in accordance with meeting my yearly goals. My yearly goals help me reach my long-term goals. I look at my goals daily and check my progress.

I believe that it is critical to have an expert in your field to help you set goals. By having Justin as my coach, it has helped me push myself in the short term and long term. At times, when I don't have the vision, I trust in his, and it allows me to reach great heights.

What is the best investment you have made either inside your career or outside of dentistry?

Continually re-evaluating what the best use of my time is. Reading books like *The 4-Hour Work Week* help me to think of the importance of my time, getting the most out of my time to allow me to be free during the remainder of my time.

As I've grown more financially successful, my currency has changed from money, to time. When I think of the costs of a purchase, it is not the money I think of, it is the time to work to earn that money that I consider. As I grow my avenues of passive income, I hope that perspective changes slightly, allowing me to rely less on working to gain income.

Dave: *I think this is an important mind shift to make once the practice of dentistry provides you a basic level of comfort and lifestyle. Time is a non-renewable resource. If we are going to avoid regrets, I feel it's critical to realize how precious time is and use it building relationships, making memories, and serving others.*

Looking back, what advice would you give yourself on the day of your dental school graduation?

Do your best clinically and just care about people.

In your opinion, what separates the top 10% of dentists from the bottom 90%?

Mindset and action. I think this is no different than the top 10% of any category of people. The top performers allow themselves to think big, and take action necessary to achieve.

I also believe that the top 1% of any category have a coach or expert that they rely on. I know some dentists in the top 10% that need to accept help and expertise if they want to reach the next level.

Justin: Agreed. I'm a believer that big accomplishments, whatever they may be, have to start with the proper mindset.

What keeps struggling dentists struggling?

Lack of proper mindset and proper action. Some have the mindset but don't take the steps necessary to achieve. Others work hard but limit themselves or their patients, due to their mindset.

What are the top 3 books every dental practice owner should read?

Sell or Be Sold by Grant Cardone
Good to Great by Jim Collins
One Minute Manager by Blanchard and Johnson

If you had to narrow it down to a couple...what traits or skills do you think are most important in running an uncommonly successful practice?

Strict love: Ability to show compassion while expecting great results, and not putting up with poor performance.

What is a skill or procedure you've added since graduating from dental school that has had a major positive impact on your practice?

Implants.

What is the best business advice you ever received?

There are so many ways to be successful and make money. You have to find what fits your style and take advantage of it.

Dave: *I feel our colleagues too often buy into a cookie-cutter approach to running a dental practice. In creating a business that "fits your style" like Derek mentions, it'll give more than just a paycheck. You can enjoy who you work with, the pace, the time away, and serving your patients by doing the procedures you most enjoy.*

What leadership advice would you give a dentist who has an ineffective culture in their practice?

You need to decide exactly what you want your practice to be like. What changes do you and your team need to make. Make the changes in yourself and expect the same of your team members.

Be quick to reprove and quick to compliment your team.

What advice would you give a dentist that is struggling with case acceptance?

First of all, do you truly believe that what you are offering the patient is the best thing for them? Do you believe it is the best use of their money? Many dentists have issues with these questions. If you don't truly believe that your dentistry should be the highest priority for your patients, start there.

Sell without selling. You can explain the needs and benefits of treatment without sounding like a salesman. Guide the patient with confidence in the right direction, but let them be in charge of making their own decision.

What marketing advice would you give a dentist that is starting out in practice ownership?

Help your new patients have excellent experiences. They will market for you, and they will help you know what is most marketable about your practice by telling you what they enjoyed most about their experience. Google reviews have been great for my practice. Almost all my new patients say that they found us on google or that after hearing about us, they checked our google reviews and decided to come in.

What do our dental patients most desire?

To hear that they don't have any cavities. jk

As little pain as possible, and finishing in as little time as possible.

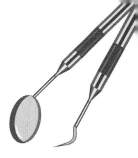

DR. DAVID HORNBROOK

Hornbrook Center for Dentistry, Clinical Director of Education at Utah Valley Dental Lab

Justin: *After taking several courses with David, I knew I wanted him included in this book. His courses are top notch, and David is a super relatable guy. We've run into each other at several dental events over the years, and I was excited when he agreed to be a part of this project.*

Background

Graduated from UCLA School of Dentistry in 1986. As materials and dentistry changed, I realized that we needed educational forums, especially live-patient treatment programs, so that dentists could master the new techniques and utilize state-of-the-art non-metal restorative materials. Founded LVI in 1995, then founded PAC~live in San Francisco. PAC~live was a live-patient anterior esthetics course that was the first course of its kind that focused on the important relationship between Function and Aesthetics. Founded the Hornbrook Group in 2002 so that we could take these courses on the road throughout North America and reach more doctors to help mentor with live-patient treatment.

Founded Clinical Mastery in 2008 as another source for doctors to understand the importance of understanding function and esthetics and created a continuum with multiple levels to meet the needs of all clinicians. Currently teaching Occlusion Courses and Functional Live-patient Esthetic Courses with Dr. Mark Montgomery.

I am also the Clinical Director of Education at Utah Valley Dental Lab in Provo, Utah, where I mentor dentists and ceramists, as both groups are better understanding the role new materials are playing in today's restorative practice and how CAD:CAM is improving the quality and options we have.

The last 20 years, I have created the Young Dentist's program though the Crown Council. I have had the opportunity to mentor over 250 Young Dentists where they attend live-patient and over-the-shoulder courses at no charge.

Please explain your style of practice (practice size, location, procedure mix, etc.)

Adult restorative private, fee-for-service with emphasis on appearance-related dentistry.

Do you have a favorite success quote or mantra?

Several...

1   You miss 100% of the shots you don't take. (Wayne Gretzky)

2   Aesthetics drives the case, and Function finishes it! (Hornbrook)

In regards to your dental career, what would you like your legacy to be, or how would you like to be remembered?

I would like to be remembered as an innovator, giver, and out-of-the-box thinker. Someone who is always willing to share with others, with the motivation being helping others achieve their personal success and fulfillment.

What does success mean to you?

To be able to say, "I love what I do," both personally and professionally and never having to say "If only, I..."

What is your morning routine (first 1–2 hrs of the day)?

Wake up at 5am, work out, walk the dog, and off to work. I start seeing patients at 6:45, so dentistry is definitely a part of the first 2 hours of every day.

What is your biggest fear?

Growing old and not being able to continue doing the things I enjoy most.

Please explain the most challenging time in your career and how you moved past it and thrived on the other side?

In 1999, I lost my right thumb in a boating accident. I am right handed and obviously this was a huge deal. Although I had the opportunity to stop practicing dentistry and collect disability, I made the commitment that this was not going to happen. Although I did have to retrain my dexterity a bit and how I held certain instruments, losing my thumb actually made me a much better dentist. I thought others might judge the quality of my clinical dentistry, so I knew I had to be a better clinician than I had ever been. It also gave me a firsthand experience how often life-changing obstacles can be overcome.

Dave: *Have you ever asked yourself what you would do tomorrow if you couldn't do dentistry? I admire how David actually improved his already superb clinical abilities. Unfortunately, I also know a few dentists that couldn't practice another day of dentistry if they wanted to. As Dr. Cory Glenn mentioned in his section, it pays to have a good disability policy. Other Titans have built up businesses that no longer require them to produce dentistry. Regardless of your plan, it pays to have one!*

What is your goal-setting process?

I am a "big picture" person, so my goals are often very broad and future based. I make lists of what steps need to be accomplished and surround myself with incredible people to help me carry out whatever it takes to get to the next step.

What is the best investment you have made either inside your career or outside of dentistry?

The very best investment has been making and nurturing incredible friendships in dentistry. It pays dividends everyday and the return is more than I could have ever imagined.

Looking back, what advice would you give yourself on the day of your dental school graduation?

Realize your vision, follow your heart, and find those that have similar visions that have blazed the paths ahead of you. Everyday I have the opportunity to counsel and mentor young dentists, and the best advice I can give is, "never say never", "stick to your dreams", and "find a mentor to follow".

In your opinion, what separates the top 10% of dentists from the bottom 90%?

Easy...their passion for what they do. Dentistry should be a "hobby" that we can make an excellent living at and not a "job" that we can't wait to retire from.

What keeps struggling dentists struggling?

Not finding the passion for what they do. I always teach "eliminate the undesirables". Those things at the morning and end of each day you regret and wish were not part of that day. This could be a certain procedure, patient, technology, philosophy...things that are keeping you from "playing" rather than "working".

Dave: *I would add team members to this. Too often we keep someone on the team that isn't a culture fit or isn't a team player. In doing so, we unintentionally undermine the potential of our top performers.*

What are the top 3 books every dental practice owner should read?

Dawson's book on Occlusion *Functional Occlusion* by Peter Dawson
Who Moved my Cheese by Ken Blanchard
Find Your Why by Simon Sinek

If you had to narrow it down to a couple...what traits or skills do you think are most important in running an uncommonly successful practice?

People skills and empathy for others. Hard to teach, but instantly recognized by all that surround you. Unwillingness to compromise.

What is a skill or procedure you've added since graduating from dental school that has had a major positive impact on your practice?

Since I started early utilizing dentistry to change people's lives with beautiful smiles, that has really not changed much over the years. Laser Dentistry and the utilization of lasers to treat periodontal disease and for closed-flap osseous procedures have taken my practice to a much higher level.

What leadership advice would you give a dentist who has an ineffective culture in their practice?

Set goals and a great vision and surround yourself with like-minded people and those that will elevate your journey to reach that vision.

What advice would you give a dentist that is struggling with case acceptance?

Treat every patient as if you are looking in a mirror. Think of dentistry as a gift you are providing; it is much easier to create value and be sincere when you are giving a life-changing gift, rather than just providing treatment. Be enthusiastic about how dentistry has changed and how these changes offer your patients exciting benefits that maybe could not be offered in the past.

What do our dental patients most desire?

To be treated as a person rather than a tooth. To be cared for, and not just operated on.

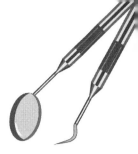

DR. CORY GLENN

Glenn Dental, Blue Sky Bio

Background

I'm Cory Glenn, and I graduated in 2008 from University of Tennessee dental school and went on to complete the 1-year AEGD residency there. I was always a lab geek throughout school—I was the guy who you could pay to set denture teeth for you or do waxups. I just really liked the hands-on aspect of dentistry and in particular, liked finding out faster or easier ways to do things.

Residency was great because I got a lot of experience in implants and larger cases, but I also had plenty of free time to tinker and just play around in the lab. After finishing, I bought a practice in a rural town of about 8,000 people in middle TN. The practice was great and we grew quickly, but one problem I realized early on was that I loved doing implants and complex cases, and yet my patients for the most part couldn't afford that type of treatment. As a result, I began figuring out a lot of ways through technology and lab techniques to be able to do big cases for patients at a high-quality level, but faster and at lower costs. That was nothing new to me...I've always been a bit of a hacker and loved just trying to learn different things.

Before dentistry, I had taught myself guitar, taxidermy, woodworking, bow-building, and a lot of other random hobbies that just caught my interest, so it was logical that I'd do the same in dentistry as well. I spent 8 years in practice before a serious medical issue rocked my world. I developed acute leukemia and had to drop everything and spend most of that year doing chemo. I recovered, thankfully, and tried for several months to go back to treating patients but still had the back problems, despite using a microscope and reduced patient loads.

Dentistry is just hard on the body, in how it forces you into so many repetitive and awkward positions. Every day I worked, I had to take narcotics at night to be able to function, and that was a dead-end solution. So, I pivoted and focused on teaching other dentists and also on the tech aspect of dentistry. This allowed me to scratch the "dentistry itch", but to also rearrange my lifestyle such that I could still work without as much pain. I'm incredibly thankful to have gone through the experience though, because it re-oriented my priorities in life and gave me a whole new appreciation for my wife and 3 daughters and all the other wonderful people in my life. I still miss clinical, but I'm really enjoying this new stage as well.

Dave: *I've known Cory for several years. He's as impressive of a person as he is a clinician. I distinctly recall where I was when I heard of his leukemia diagnosis. I was shocked. It looked at first that it might be a terminal illness. I recall chatting with him via Facebook one day when he was still in the hospital. He asked what I was doing that day, and I said I'm going out skiing with my family. He said, "When you get up on that mountain, check out the view and breathe that air in. Breathe it in deep." I often think about his challenge to me. To this day, it reminds me to be grateful for all I have.*

Please explain your style of practice (practice size, location, procedure mix, etc.)

At one time, I had a high-volume, mostly insurance-based, rural practice with all the bells and whistles and technology you could want. My staff was 2 assistants, 2 hygienists, and 2 administrators, with my wife doing all the books and behind-the-scenes work. We were very successful and I truly loved it.

However, since I've had to retire from clinical dentistry due to back issues, I've shifted into teaching and tech development for Blue Sky Bio. Nowadays, you'll find me in a new facility a few blocks away from my old practice that I purchased and renovated to specifically accommodate my new job. I really wanted to build something to function as an office away from home that I would enjoy going to, as well as a teaching facility. Obviously, since I do tech development, there's lots of technology...scanners, 3D printers, microscopes, lab equipment, etc. But I'm also a redneck, so there's deer heads on the wall, rustic furniture, big screen TVs, and guitars on the wall. I have exercise equipment and stand-up desks that I custom made to keep me moving and prevent my back from flaring up as I work.

Any given hour in a day, you may find me 3D printing jaws, answering customer service emails, experimenting with new restorative techniques, or doing kettlebell swings and pull-ups. And if I get overwhelmed or have trouble concentrating, I'll take a 10-minute break and crank some tunes to play along with on guitar. It's a cool place to work and give courses in—a big man cave. In a lot of ways, I'm busier than I was even in clinical practice, but I still enjoy it.

Do you have a favorite success quote or mantra?

Like many dentists I meet, I am a gunner. I don't do moderation well and I tend to obsess on one thing, often at the expense of other more important things. I like the Dali Lama's quote about man to remind myself to keep that in check:

> *[Man] sacrifices his health in order to make money. Then he sacrifices money to recuperate his health. And then he is so anxious about the future that he does not enjoy the present; the result being that he does not live in the present or the future; he lives as if he is never going to die, and then dies having never really lived.*

In regards to your dental career, what would you like your legacy to be, or how would you like to be remembered?

I want to have made dentistry more affordable and more accessible to both the clinicians carrying it out and patients receiving it. I got so sick of everyone in dentistry wanting $300 a month from me and making my life ever increasingly complicated. I believe we can simplify and drastically lower the cost of dentistry by utilizing technology. Not some closed system that costs hundreds of thousands of dollars, but rather, something that a dentist in an impoverished country could use just like a wealthy dentist could.

Take surgical guides...who would have thought 10 years ago when it cost $500 to get a guided surgery stent that we would be able to now plan it in house and 3D print it in a couple of hours for $20 total? The same will happen and *is* happening with things like ortho, dentures, and digital restorative. I want to be part of what makes it happen.

What does success mean to you?

That those who are closest to me know I love them and would do anything for them and that my colleagues and community would be able to say I added value to their lives.

What is your morning routine (first 1–2 hrs of the day)?

I wake up, shower, and have coffee. I always take my 3 daughters to school and then it's off to my facility to get in a quick, 30 minute workout. I usually listen to a podcast or audiobook as I do it and then try to start to work by 9 at the latest.

Please explain the most challenging time in your career and how you moved past it and thrived on the other side?

Definitely my cancer diagnosis at the end of 2015. We were at our prime and everything professionally was going perfect...my practice was thriving; I was doing the kind of dentistry I loved; and my speaking career was just on the verge of taking off. However, I'd achieved all that at the expense of many other things. I had been way too focused on work and not on my family, health, diet, or exercise, and by the end of that year I felt miserable.

I began coming home every day with excruciating back pain and exhaustion and other strange symptoms. The terrible back pain and hand cramps that were hindering me professionally finally drove me to the doctor, and that's when they discovered I had acute leukemia. I was a wreck, and it suddenly became clear to me that all that stuff didn't matter at all, and the only thing that did ultimately matter in my life was relationships.

In that regard, cancer was the best thing that ever happened to me. Through 8 months of chemo and lots of support from my family, friends, and staff, I fully recovered from the leukemia; but I was not able to overcome the chronic back pain, which is why I had to shift my focus away from clinical dentistry. The interesting thing, though, is that I was pretty public throughout that process, and my speaking career absolutely exploded after that. God really provided for us and even though the clinical door closed, I had a lot of other doors open.

What is your goal-setting process?

I typically write down a big list of goals on Dec 31 and get all pumped about crushing it...and then I lose the list within a couple days and just wing it. I'm terrible at that stuff.

What is the best investment you have made either inside your career or outside of dentistry?

Disability insurance. It's one of those things you hope you never need, but I had some people wisely tell me to max it out at every opportunity as your income increases. I'm so glad I followed their advice, because life would be a lot more difficult without it now. There are very few things as productive as being a practicing dentist.

Looking back, what advice would you give yourself on the day of your dental school graduation?

Chill out! You don't have to conquer the world by tomorrow afternoon.

In your opinion, what separates the top 10% of dentists from the bottom 90%?

Well, it depends on in what category…if we're talking top-10% earners, I'd say communication skills. Top 10% in job satisfaction—then maybe ability to surround themselves with a great team that helps bear the burdens of practice. Top 10% in clinical excellence would be an unwavering commitment to do it right, regardless of how much time it takes them or what they're going to be paid. In my experience, these things rarely all coexist within a single practitioner.

What keeps struggling dentists struggling?

The inability to adapt and change.

Dave: *The technological innovations are currently hard to keep up with. Commitment to CE and implementation of the new technology into practice is going to be increasingly important for career success.*

What are the top 3 books every dental practice owner should read?

When Breath Becomes Air by Paul Kalanithi
The Little Book of Common Sense Investing by John Bogle
The Bible

If you had to narrow it down to a couple...what traits or skills do you think are most important in running an uncommonly successful practice?

The best all-around docs I know have a knack for hiring great staff and then training them and incentivizing them to perform. They get the most from their teams, which in turn frees the doctor to focus on patient care.

What is a skill or procedure you've added since graduating from dental school that has had a major positive impact on your practice?

Dental implants and photography.

What is the best business advice you ever received?

Don't care more about the patient's teeth than they do. Not everyone deserves or even needs teeth, so that takes a lot of pressure off.

What leadership advice would you give a dentist who has an ineffective culture in their practice?

First, be sure you're not a jerk; that may be the source of toxic team atmosphere. Then, identify and eliminate members of the team that may be. Life is too short and dentistry itself is too difficult to add in more drama.

Dave: *Motivational speaker Jim Rohn famously said that we are the average of the 5 people we spend the most time with. For dentists, the 5 people you spend the most time with are usually in your office. Select them wisely.*

What advice would you give a dentist that is struggling with case acceptance?

You gotta be confident talking to patients. If you aren't confident recommending it, they smell it from a mile away and won't do it.

What marketing advice would you give a dentist that is starting out in practice ownership?

Get a camera and take pictures of everything. It will elevate the standards of your work and also provide you a ton of free marketing material for sharing on the office walls, social media, and advertising.

What do our dental patients most desire?

The same thing we all want...perfection at no cost! Hence, the difficulty in being a dentist!

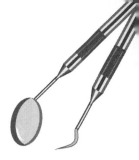

DR. MARK COSTES

Dental Success Institute, The Dentalpreneur Podcast

Dave: *Mark accomplishes more in a month than most people do in a year. I've spent time with him at many conferences. He has seemingly endless energy to engage the audience and in helping them gain a competitive advantage. Most recently, we've worked together (along with many other generous dentists) on building the Dental Success Network. We've both had significant career struggles and are committed to helping the next generation of dentists "breathe a little easier".*

Background

Dr. Mark Costes is far from a typical dentist and dental coach. During his career, he has been able to start or acquire 14 successful dental practices during some of the profession's most challenging times.

Dr. Costes is founder of the Dental Success Institute, a company committed to helping dentists to achieve their full potential, while recapturing their passion for dentistry. He is also the founder of the Horizon Schools of Dental Assisting, which has experienced explosive growth and has expanded to over 180 locations throughout the United

States. Dr. Costes is the International and #1 Amazon Best Selling Author of the book *Pillars of Dental Success*.

His internet radio show, *The Dentalpreneur Podcast*, now has listenership from 149 countries worldwide. Mark is committed to community involvement and serves as chairman of the board at the Yavapai Big Brothers and Big Sisters organization and is the founder and chairman of Dental Outreach International. Mark and his wife, Leslie, have 3 sons: Bryce, Brendan, Brady, and their dog Bear. They live in Prescott, AZ. Mark enjoys any and all outdoor activities as well as coaching his son's soccer and baseball teams.

Do you have a favorite success quote or mantra?

We don't use the word overwhelm in our offices anymore, because we all are feeling that we're overwhelmed, and we're overly stressed, and kind of tapped out emotionally, and even physically as far as how hard we are all working, so we don't use that word anymore. We're more focused on gratitude. So, my new favorite quote is, "The struggle ends when gratitude begins." And that's by Neil Donald Walsh.

I think there are so many layers to that quote, but it doesn't take a genius to realize that in most cases, we're all very, very fortunate to be in the position that we're in, especially as professionals as far as dentists go. We're also fortunate to be in the top 3% of all educated people in the world.

In regards to your dental career, what would you like your legacy to be, or, how would you want to be remembered?

Wow. That one can go a lot of different directions. I believe that—I have to believe this, and that is that I'm making the profession better by helping people to navigate around the mistakes that I've personally made. I've made so many mistakes as far as work-life balance, and mistakes with the way that I've run my businesses, the way that I've treated employees in the past. So many mistakes.

I believe that if I can share that with our profession and help them to avoid some of the big mistakes that I've made, that almost cost me dearly in my life, in my personal life and my business life, that would be a great legacy. So, that is the way I go into every single consultation, and while working with every single dentist that I work with, I want to make their life better. I want to decrease their stress and increase the amount of time that they get to spend doing things that they love to do.

In addition to that, our new focus for our group of dental practices is, we really have a mission-centered approach now, where we want to deliver as much access to dentistry for people that can't afford it as we can. We've created a new organization called Dental Outreach International, where we're helping people all over the world to get access to dental care.

Those are just a couple of things. I want people to remember me for helping them to navigate some of the mistakes that I made, and to improve the quality of their lives—their practice lives and their personal lives—and to provide a lot of access to dental care to people that can't afford it around the world.

What does success mean to you?

It's a tough question because, depending on the time of day and the day, it changes. But really, success to me means that I'm living what I believe is my purpose, that I'm making the world a better place, and now I'm serving the people that are most important to me, the best that I can. I want to be the best husband, son, father, friend, mentor that I can possibly be. And if I could live by those ideals, then I lived a successful life.

What is your morning routine?

I have a very tangible morning routine. It usually takes about 90 minutes. I'm an early riser, and always have been. First thing I do when

I wake up is I have a 16-ounce glass of water; I chug it. I pop out of bed, and I go right to the gym. I have a very, very regimented routine that usually takes less than 20 minutes in the gym. Then I do some sort of quiet reflection. Sometimes it's guided meditation. Sometimes it's watching a motivational video. Sometimes it's just taking a walk in the woods. Quiet reflection time.

Then I do something creative, where I'm either writing a blog post, recording a podcast, writing a chapter for my next book, something creative. Then I set my agenda for the day. I figure out what it is that are my top priorities for the day. I try to stack those priorities earlier in the day, so that most of my most important things are done before 10:30 in the morning, and then I go about my day.

What is your biggest fear?

My biggest fear is not living up to my full potential. Not realizing it, and not living my purpose. There have been times in my life where I strayed from what really mattered, and my priorities got out of whack. That is my biggest fear, to go down that road and not realize that it's happening. Not living up to my full potential and not serving the way that I know that I can.

Can you explain a challenging time in your career and how you moved past it and thrived on the other side?

Probably one of the toughest times in my career, from the outside looking in, might have looked to other people that it was the best time of my career. The first 7 years of my dental career, I built 6 very successful dental practices. I had a goal of being a multiple practice owner, and I had a very specific income goal in my mind, and I had achieved that pretty early in my career, when I was still in my mid-30s.

However, the unintended negative backstory was that my personal life was spinning out of control. While I was focusing all of my energy and bandwidth on building the business, I was neglecting all of the most important people in my life. I was neglecting my wife, and my kids, and my parents, and I wasn't a good friend; I wasn't a good boss. Almost all at once, I realized that although I was a very successful business person at the time and I had hit my monetary goals, that it was time to reset.

At that point, I sold 4 of my 6 practices, and that's exactly what I did; I reset. I reset my priorities. I redefined my non-negotiables, and I prioritized my personal life, and figured out a better way to run my businesses so that I wasn't the bottleneck in all of my businesses. That decreased the amount of stress on my relationships and on me personally.

That was probably the most difficult time in my professional life. I'm happy to say that since I've done the exercise of reprioritizing, the business continues to grow, and I'm doing it the right way now, by being true to my non-negotiables.

What is your goal setting process?

I set goals typically several times per year. For each of my practices and my businesses, we have monetary goals in place. We have growth goals in place. We have overhead goals in place. That typically takes place...the goal-setting process usually happens twice per year, one at the midpoint of the year and one at the beginning of the year.

We set quarterly goals through the year. Then I have personal development goals as well, things that I want to—character traits that I want to develop, experiences that I want to have, and things that I want to do, things that I want to be, do, have. Business goals are in there as well, but personal development and relationship goals are in there as well.

What's the best investment you've made, either inside your career or outside of dentistry?

I always say that the greatest information in the world you can pick up for less than $25, and those are books. Of all of my mentors that

I have had, some of them I've met, some of them I haven't, some of them are alive, some of them are dead. I am a voracious consumer of biographies, of business books, of nonfiction books about relationships, psychology, leadership, business.

My best investment that I've made in myself is taking the time to consume that material, and then obviously, the $25 that it costs to purchase any one of those. I'm currently reading several biographies and several business books as we speak. All told, some of the best material that I've read, less than 100 bucks for all of that great material.

Looking back, what advice would you give yourself on the day that you graduated from dental school?

I think if I was looking back, I would say, "Hey man, take it easy. Make sure that in your pursuit of financial goals and success, that you're remembering to prioritize your personal relationships. Make sure that you define what it is that you're really here for, and the reason that you're doing all of this. Don't get lost in the busyness of trying to create something—some sort of financial success."

Dave: *If you consider yourself a driven dentist, stop and read that one more time!*

In your opinion, what separates the top 10% of dentists from the other 90%?

This question goes deep for me. I truly believe that people that have the ability to have a clear vision of where they want to go really separate the ultra-achievers from the mediocre. What I mean by that is, if you can identify exactly where it is that you want to be, and reverse engineer the path, I believe that's what most of the high achievers in the world have been able to do.

A clear vision first, and then reverse engineer each step on how to get there. Surround yourself with people that are smarter than yourself, and people that fill the gaps for areas that aren't your strong points. For instance, if you are not great at tech, you need to surround yourself with people that are.

If you are not necessarily the best speaker or leader, you need to surround yourself with people that are good at that, and that can mentor you to get better at that. If you are not the most organized person in the world, you need to surround yourself with a staff that keeps you organized.

If you have a tendency to overbook yourself, then you need somebody on staff that can help you schedule your life in the most efficient manner. I would say that being able to have a clear vision, and work backwards from that vision, and surrounding yourself with people that are smarter than you in certain areas and that plug the holes for your weaknesses, I think that's what successful people do that average people don't.

What keeps struggling dentists struggling?

Unfortunately, I get to see a lot of dentists that are frustrated and struggling. One of the things that we work on every single day is to help them pull themselves out of difficult times. I believe that people that struggle have trouble with perspective, and get distracted by details, oftentimes. There are some people that obsess over the smallest detail, and I think that dentists by nature are very detailed oriented; but if you don't have the ability to step back and say, "Okay, this is one tiny part of a bigger problem," and the ability to appraise the problem for really what it is, those are the people that get stuck and don't progress in life or in their careers.

What are the top 3 books every dental practice owner should read?

The E-Myth Revisited by Michael Gerber
Extreme Ownership by Jocko Willink and Leif Babin
The Four Disciplines of Execution by Sean Covey

If you had to narrow it down to just a couple, what traits or skills do you think are the most important in running an uncommonly successful dental practice?

I think it's the ability to build rapport and relationships with both your team, and your patients. Also leadership, because you can have the best systems in the world, you can have the best business background in the world; but if you don't have the ability to attract and retain the right people on your team, and have the leadership ability to lead them, then all of the best systems in the world are useless.

Notice I didn't say anything about your clinical ability. I think clinical ability is a distant third to those two traits.

What is a skill or a procedure that you've added since graduating from dental school that has had a major positive impact on your practice?

I'm going to have to take that back to a previous question where I was saying that I had those 6 very successful dental practices; but I was working 80 hours a week, and I didn't have a good quality of life, and I was the bottleneck in all of those practices.

The reason that was so stressful—because there are people that have far more than 6 successful dental practices and do it just fine—the reason that I was so stressed and inefficient during that time was because I did not have good systems in place at the practice level, at each individual practice level. I would have to say that one skill, or trait, that I've picked up since then is the ability to lead a team, and to put systems in place and hold that team accountable.

That really is the number one thing that's been able to separate me from other dental groups, and has improved the quality of my life since graduating, and even more so, after that first 7 years until now.

What did you do to develop your leadership confidence?

Leadership is a very, very difficult thing, right? I don't believe that most good leaders are born. I believe that that is developed over time, and I believe that you have to be intentional about building that muscle. I believe that leadership is like a muscle. You have to practice, and you have to develop that over time. I believe that, at a base level, there is lots of great free content out there; you have to immerse yourself and model some of the greatest leaders in the world.

I have read dozens of books on leadership. I have watched countless videos, YouTube videos, and consumed other types of content that are dedicated to improving your leadership ability. I believe that a big part about leadership is being able to motivate and keep things in perspective. There are a lot of resources out there, to help you to develop into a bigger—a better leader.

What's the best business advice you've ever received?

I think probably the best business advice that I've ever received is that—it goes back to leadership. You've got to be able to lead, inspire your team of people. You have to be able to assemble, retain, and inspire a great team in order to be successful in any business venture.

What leadership advice would you give a dentist who has an ineffective culture in their practice?

It honestly is a matter of getting the right people sitting in the right seats. You have to have the right people on board that work well together, that care about the overall health of the business. As a leader, you have to be able to foster that culture. You have to live that culture and emanate that culture.

What advice would you give a dentist who is struggling with case acceptance?

Case acceptance is all about the relationship. Case acceptance is about building trust in a very short period of time. If you have a new patient sitting in the chair, they have gone through a series of touches with your office. They have responded to some sort of external marketing campaign, or they've been referred by a friend; they've called your office, and made an appointment. The office called to confirm; now they're sitting in your dental chair.

They sat in your reception area. They were brought back. X-rays were taken. All told, they've had contact with your office maybe less than an hour. Then you go in there, and you start speaking with a patient for 15 to 20 minutes, before you start giving your case presentation. At some point, you are going to have to build enough trust in this patient, in this doctor-patient relationship, that they are going to believe what you say, and they're going to say yes to treatment.

At its root level, you have to remember—as the dentist, as the person giving the case presentation—that it all comes down to trust, rapport, and relationship. The faster you can get to that point, by whatever means, the better chance you're going to have at closing that case. Make sure that the conversation is about the patient. You don't get lost in a bunch of vocabulary that the patient doesn't understand. Bring the conversation down to their level and try to tie it into a personal example.

"I would suggest this for my mother, or my grandfather, or my dad, and for the following reasons..." Build trust as quickly as possible. Build that rapport and relationship as quickly as possible, and you'll see your case acceptance increase dramatically.

What marketing advice would you give a dentist that is starting out in practice ownership?

First of all, make sure that you are aware of the sources of new patients, the current sources of new patients. Then figure out what your ad budget is going to be, or what your marketing budget is going to be. I usually suggest something around 5% for a seasoned practice, and sometimes about 10% of revenue for a brand-new practice.

Now, you can allocate that budget in a lot of different ways. What works in one market isn't necessarily going to work in a different market. I have seen that it's very important to have a good web presence. Spending a little bit of money on SEO and having a good quality website is very important. It is basically what the majority of the people are going to check before they decide to make an appointment at your office.

I have seen that Ad Words are a good way to spend money, but it doesn't work in every market. When you're looking at the traditional methods of advertising—we have radio, TV, print ads, direct mail, SEO, Google Ad Words—it really comes down to testing and tracking.

For instance, if you notice after a couple of months that you're getting zero patients coming in from your print ad, you know you need to change the message or the offer on your print ad, or you need to eliminate it completely and reallocate your funds in a different area.

Testing and tracking is probably the biggest advice I could give someone, because like I said, one method in one market isn't necessarily going to carry over to another, so it's very difficult to give blanket marketing advice to every single practice out there.

What do our dental patients most desire?

I think that dental patients are no different than human beings in general. I mean, dental patients are human beings, and what they want is to be heard, and they want to be cared for by somebody that has their best interests at heart. If you could convey that to your patients, you're not going to have an attrition problem.

If you could convey that they mean something to you—they're not just a tooth, they're not just a number, that you care about their overall health, and their well-being, and their comfort—then they'll stay with you forever.

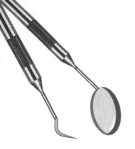

DR. PAUL ETCHISON

Nelson Ridge Family Dental,
Dental Practice Heroes Podcast, Author

Justin: Dave and I have both been on Paul's podcast, and we think you'll really enjoy this interview, because it's raw and filled with some great pearls.

Background

Dr. Paul Etchison is a practicing dentist in New Lenox, IL. He is also the founder of the *Dental Practice Heroes Podcast*, the author of *Dental Practice Hero: From Ordinary Practice to Extraordinary Experience*, and a national speaker.

He resides in Frankfort, IL with his wife and 2 daughters. Dr. Etchison was born in the city of Joliet, Illinois. He graduated from the University of Illinois Urbana-Champaign, with a Bachelors of Science in Advertising. Dr. Etchison then attended the University Of Illinois College Of Dentistry, where he was awarded his Doctor of Dental Surgery Degree along with a Bachelors of Science in Dentistry in 2009.

In 2013, he was awarded Fellowship into the International Congress of Oral Implantologists. In 2015, he was awarded Fellowship into the

Academy of General Dentistry. He is an active board member for the Chicago Chapter of the AGD.

Please explain your style of practice (practice size, location, procedure mix, etc.)

I opened a scratch start 6 years ago in a suburb of Chicago about 40 miles from the city. We have been predominantly PPO since the beginning. We are beginning to gain insurance dependence, but we are still about 80% PPO. I hope to reduce this tremendously in the near future. Last year (2017), we collected $2.85MM and this year I think we will hit $3.3MM.

We are a fast-paced office. We are big on efficiency, but we stress our culture and teamwork over everything else. I have been blessed with 23 employees and have had zero turnover since our original open date.

I perform almost all speciality procedures personally (i.e. ortho, endo, surgical extractions, implants, botox, etc.)

We are a split-shifted office open from 7am to 8pm, 4 nights a week (Monday through Thursday) and 7–3 on Friday.

I see patients 3 days a week (22 hours) and my associate does 5 days (about 40 hours).

Do you have a favorite success quote or mantra?

"He who walks with integrity walks securely, he who takes crooked paths will be found out."

—PROVERBS 10:9

If we always do things for the right reasons, we will always be rewarded and will never feel guilt. Keeping our word as golden should be one of our highest priorities.

In regards to your dental career, what would you like your legacy to be, or how would you like to be remembered?

I want my legacy to be about helping others achieve the lifestyle that currently I enjoy. While income is a part of that, time is much more important to me. I want dentists to realize that dentistry is really hard on us mentally and physically, and that we can enjoy great livings on only 3 or fewer days a week. I graduated undergrad as an advertising major. That background has given me a special lens to view customer service and patient experience through. I want to share what has worked so well for me, so that other dentists, private practicing dentists in particular, can enjoy the same benefit I do, working a 3-day work week and taking 12 weeks vacation each year. I think we are all rat racing to retirement and in the process, missing our entire lives. I want to change this in our profession.

I also want to remembered as someone who helped another dentist create a great team culture that works together so well, that running the practice becomes much less stressful. I think I do this very well at my practice, and I want to share it with our colleagues.

What does success mean to you?

Success to me means having relationships and experiences that matter to me outside of the office, all the while enjoying my time in the office, because the culture and systems allow me to be highly productive while I am there and while I am not.

Success is being able to choose the way you practice. For instance, money is not very important to me anymore; my time and stress level take priority. I have been scaling my clinical days back and relaxing my days a bit, because I no longer feel the need to produce at the level I am used to. Don't get me wrong, I am still producing at a level of $1100–$1250 a hour, but I am not running around like crazy on the verge of a heart attack anymore.

Justin: Success means a lot of different things to different people, but I really liked Paul's definitions. One of my related definitions of success is very similar, which is, being able to choose the way you live. More than money, I want to choose how I live, how I spend my time, and who I get to spend it with.

What is your morning routine (first 1–2 hrs of the day)?

Two of my clinical days begin at 7am, so I don't do much more than wake, shower, and go to work. On my later day, I will lift weights and try to cross things off of my never-ending to do list.

I always choose one or two "frogs" to start with. These are always the things that tend to sit on the to do list for a long time because I don't want to do them. I get these done first before the other easier things, because I know if I don't, I will spend time crossing off easier, more enjoyable tasks and never get to the "frogs". I have been doing the 5-minute journal since January and have really enjoyed starting my day with positivity and gratitude.

On my days off, I always work out first thing.

I don't meditate, nor do I stand in the mirror and tell myself I am worthy and valuable. I just work out, and usually that's just weights, because I hate cardio.

What is your biggest fear?

My biggest fear is that people will conclude that I have no idea what I am talking about or that I am a really bad clinician. I constantly feel the pressure of the *imposter syndrome*. I am not sure if it is lack of confidence or just human nature, but I struggle with this. I know in my heart that I have something worth sharing, that I have been very successful in my practice, and that my work is clinically excellent; yet self-doubt tends to rear its head from time to time.

Dave: *So common. Yet, few are courageous enough to admit it! Many dentists are running themselves into the ground simply trying to "Be enough". If you struggle with this, read the next section to get some clues on how to make the shift from constantly chasing significance to finding joy in the day to day.*

Please explain the most challenging time in your career and how you moved past it and thrived on the other side?

The most challenging point in my career was about 2 years into my startup. I had just paid off both my cars and all of my student loans. The practice was doing really well and I wasn't exactly prepared to be having the income I was experiencing. I'll explain a little further...

My whole life, I was always very stressed out, always waiting for the next thing so that I could be happy. I was waiting to accomplish the next goal, or to get through this busy portion of my life so that I could finally start living.

What I realized, was that after the practice was a success, I had checked off all the obstacles that were getting in the way of my being happy. I had graduated college, conquered dental school, and owned my own successful practice that was financially sound; I had a nice car, a nice house, I was married with one daughter at the time...there wasn't anything left for me to check off except for retirement, which was still quite a ways away.

I got to the point I had been diving towards my whole life and realized I still wasn't happy. So if I reached all my goals, and I wasn't happy, what the hell was wrong with me?

I had to come to grips that I had an entirely wrong thought process my whole life. I had to realize that it wasn't in the reaching of goals but the process that I was supposed to be enjoying. I finally found that I had everything I needed to be happy the whole time, not just after reaching my big goals.

I had to change the way I thought and how I worked. I was working too much and my relationships were suffering. I went from 2 weeks of vacation that year to 8 weeks immediately. I was seeing a therapist that helped me talk through some issues. I started setting some goals that weren't financial or career oriented.

I can't say that I still don't struggle with taking on too much, or being too career focused, but I am much better than I was, and I'm at a great place in my life with my family right now. I wouldn't change a thing. For if I had not gone through that process, I may still be chasing goals and dreams that, once materialized, would be unfulfilling.

What is your goal-setting process?

I love writing down my goals on paper, reverse engineering them, and then writing the steps on a whiteboard in my office. I do this for my personal and professional goals. To me, no goal is real unless it is on my white board. Once I get clear about what I want to do, I can then get clear about the steps I need to take to get there, and the whiteboard is my visual reminder every day to at least get one thing accomplished that moves the needle closer to where I want to be.

I try to enjoy the journey more, because as I have explained previously, I tend to want to rush towards the end goal and miss the beauty in its manifestation.

Dave: *If you don't own a whiteboard (or two), get yourself one and start getting all those thoughts bouncing around in your head onto the whiteboard. It's magical what can come out of a quiet room with a whiteboard and some dry erase markers after 20 min!*

What is the best investment you have made either inside your career or outside of dentistry?

The best investment I have ever made was being a CE junky from graduation. I have always enjoyed continuing to learn. I am a big reader of business, achievement, personal betterment, and communication books.

I feel like my continued dedication to learning has given me the edge I need to be very successful. One of my favorite quotes is from Ralph Waldo Emerson: "Each man I meet in my walks is my superior in one way or another." Meaning that I can learn something from every single person I meet. I love traveling for CE and getting together with other dentists to talk about what is working at their practices and in their lives. I don't do it as much as I used to before I had 2 kids, but I still get away for a distant CE at least 4–5 times a year.

There is no better investment than investing in your skills and business knowledge.

Looking back, what advice would you give yourself on the day of your dental school graduation?

Just to do your best all the time and accept that not everything is going to turn out perfect. When it comes to clinical dentistry, or the situations at the practice, be accepting of things that are less than perfect.

I have stressed out and poured so much energy into cases and things that have gone wrong at the practice. I've thought long about things while being with my family, while laying in bed trying to fall asleep, and even in the middle of the night not being able to fall back asleep. I used to believe that everything could and should be perfect; I have learned to loosen up lately, which has been good.

I think a lot of the time we as dentists are trained to be perfectionists, and when our expectations are so high, it's often that we don't meet them. This makes us feel like we failed, when in reality, we probably are doing very well.

I think we should go for acceptable. What that means will be different for each and every person. I am not advocating for treating patients or people badly—what is "acceptable" for me, I feel, is still better than 95% of the dentists out there—but I am no longer stressing myself out over things that weren't "perfect" or when someone on my team makes a mistake.

In your opinion, what separates the top 10% of dentists from the bottom 90%?

Intentionality. That's all! Be intentional about everything: your learning, your systems, your team, your culture, your patient experience, your procedures, your goals, your life, your family, etc. Get clear about what you want in all of the areas of your being, and then execute. The difference between the top and bottom is that the top is intentional about what they want, and then they put in the time and mental energy to get that shit done.

I would also add CE and reading books, because if you don't hear new ideas or hear about what is possible, you are stuck.

Third, I would stress that having a great team is the foundation of any solid practice, and that the all-star team stems from the leader. The people aren't just found; they are developed and cared for.

Dave: *All those things Paul mentioned are going to happen by design or by default. Default is a crap shoot and rarely positive. May as well design them (your learning, your systems, your team, your culture, your patient experience, your procedures, your goals, your life, your family, etc.) exactly how you want them. Right?!*

What keeps struggling dentists struggling?

Most dentists are blamers. They don't take responsibility for what is going on in their lives and in their practices. Dentists need to look at every issue, every little thing that happens at the practice as well as in their lives, and take 100% responsibility for it.

Struggling dentists believe they are victims of their environments and everything that is negative is outside of their control. This is a defeating attitude. Once a dentist looks at everything through the lens of making everything their problem and responsibility, they are empowered to change it. If they do not have that attitude, they cannot be a good leader; and without a good leader, a practice will always struggle.

What are the top 3 books every dental practice owner should read?

Making Money is Killing Your Business by Chuck Blakeman
E-Myth Revisited by Michael Gerber
*The Subtle Art of Not Giving a F*ck* by Mark Manson

If you had to narrow it down to a couple...what traits or skills do you think are most important in running an uncommonly successful practice?

Three things: First, communication. Communicating with your team and with your patients. Just like a good marriage, a good practice has good communication between all involved parties. The practice needs to be a safe place where people are free to make mistakes without judgement. If you criticize or belittle your team, you will create a culture in which team members will only try to do the very least to not get in trouble. If you create an environment that is safe, your team will have the confidence to take the lead, all the while knowing that if they screw up, you won't make them feel awful about it.

Leadership is critical as well. Leading your team to where you want to go as well as leading your patients to what you want them to choose. Sales is in essence leadership. You are selling your team on your vision just like you are selling your patient on your recommendations.

Lastly, integrity. Have integrity in everything you do. Make your word mean something by always following through on every commitment you make, big or small. Always do what you say you are going to do, as well as do it for the right reason. The right reason can never be selfish. It has to contribute some good to the world. If you act with integrity, you might be able to lead a team; if you don't, you're dead before you even begin.

What is a skill or procedure you've added since graduating from dental school that has had a major positive impact on your practice?

Hard to say...I really enjoy ortho, implants, and molar endo. They are still fun and challenging to me after nearly 10 years of being a dentist. However, if I had to pick one skill, it would be the ability to implement block scheduling. Nothing has allowed my office to produce the way it does like block scheduling. I can't imagine scheduling any other way. I honestly feel it is the best.

What is the best business advice you ever received?

That you need to take time to run the business, not just work inside of it. Much like the theme of the E-Myth, you need to have time in the practice with your team that doesn't involve seeing patients. You need to train and communicate with your team so that you can grow your practice and be the best you can be.

The times in my practice life that have been the worst (upset staff, upset patients, burn out) have always been when I haven't spent a lot of time in the practice running and managing the business. Usually in the summertime, because I am traveling or playing golf. Once I get back into the business and start communicating with my team, planning, and leading—the problems at the practice go away, and our culture and morale improves. The business needs my leadership and direction to continue to be as successful as it is. People can talk about self-managed teams all they want—I do believe in that principle—but I still think the team needs that regular infusion of energy from the leader to continue performing.

Dave: *I can't tell you how many dentists I've talked to who have told me that everything got better in their lives when they made an effort to be in the practice fewer days. It gives them time for rest and relaxation, thinking time, time to work on the business. Therefore they are hyper focused and super productive on those days they are with patients.*

What leadership advice would you give a dentist who has an ineffective culture in their practice?

Communicate with your team! Start there! The next week, take each team member to your office to have what I call a "no-agenda meeting". This is a one-on-one talk to ask what is going well, what is not going well, what we can do to improve, and anything else you want to ask.

Then you need to treat all this information as confidential, just like if your best friend was telling you a secret. Never break the trust of your team, because they will give you all the information you need to improve your practice. If you break their trust, they won't feel comfortable sharing anything with you. Same as if you get defensive. Remember, there is no need to defend yourself, because everything is your responsibility. So own it!

Then be clear with your team what you want the practice to stand for and where you want it go. They then can decide if they will buy into that or not. Sometimes it is hard to change people and culture, and people need to be fired. If that is the case, you just need to make sure that you are clear with the new hires about your vision and what you want. Eventually you will have a team full of people who are with you instead of against you. I will add that I feel like most of us have a lot of stars on our team and we often fire too early instead of developing and training. There is no right or wrong and every practice is different; I just feel in my opinion, we often give up on team members before we are ever clear about our expectations and what we want them to do. The problem is, that most dentists are not intentional or clear about what they want in the first place. That would be a great place to put some energy.

Most importantly, you have to walk the walk. You need to model exactly what you want from your team. Nothing will be important to them if it is not first important to you.

What advice would you give a dentist that is struggling with case acceptance?

Take some case acceptance CE. Bruce Baird, Paul Homoly, Chris Phelps, etc. Listen to my podcast; it is a common theme on most of my podcasts. Read some books on communication and likability.

Realize that case acceptance depends on the entire patient experience from phone call all the way to leaving the practice after the visit, not just the words you use. It's also important to be confident and authentic.

I would add that the most important thing I have ever changed to increase my case acceptance, is to get to know the patient personally before discussing anything clinical. People want to buy from people they like. Find some common ground with the patient and get to know them a little better.

What marketing advice would you give a dentist that is starting out in practice ownership?

Your best marketing is creating such an amazing experience for your patients, that they tell all their friends and family about you. My startup had amazing growth and still continues to (80–120 np's a month). We do dabble in marketing from time to time (PPC, mailers, etc.), but for the most part, our growth is due to creating "raving fans" who refer people to us.

What do our dental patients most desire?

To be understood and listened to. Every patient should not get the same treatment plan; it needs to be specific to them based on their goals and values. The only way to know their goals and values for their oral health is to ask. It may seem weird, but ask your patient what their goals for their mouth and smile are.

Someone whose goals are, "I want to have the best dental health possible," is going to get a very different treatment plan than someone who says, "I just don't want to lose any more teeth and only fix what is necessary."

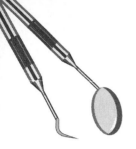

DR. NATHAN JEAL

Avant Dental Care, Follow-App, Dental Authority Marketing

Background

Born and raised in Vancouver, BC. Studied in Quebec and Winnipeg. Graduate of University of Manitoba 2011. Bought and sold 5 practices since then. Currently have 2 practices, one urban and one semi-rural. Went from doing zero orthodontic and cosmetic cases to doing over 100 a year after studying marketing principles and applying them to digital ads. Spend one week a year providing free dental care in Jamaica where the ratio of pop:dentist is 20,000:1.

Have created the only connection to infusionsoft that exists, linking a web and mobile app to the most powerful automated marketing platform anywhere. My creation, Follow-App (follow-app.io) is the digital prescription to cure poor case acceptance. All with the push of a button.

Co-founded Dental Authority Marketing (DAM) to provide authority marketing to select dentists across North America. Our marketing strategies use digital, print, radio, and TV media to establish local expert status. DAM delivers prequalified leads to dentist clients who want to transform their life and practice.

Dave: *Nate is one of those guys who can seemingly collapse time. He and his wife BT are both dentists and friends of mine. I'm amazed at what they've accomplished in their short careers. Nate is a perpetual student of business, marketing, sales, and clinical dentistry. His successes come from his decisiveness and the ability to intersect those diverse skills he's always enhancing.*

Please explain your style of practice (practice size, location, procedure mix, etc.)

One day a week of consults, only 2 days a week hands-on treatment, primarily solving patient frustration with broken, crooked, or missing teeth or loose dentures.

Do you have a favorite success quote or mantra?

> *"There is nothing more unequal than the equal treatment of unequals."*
>
> —VINCE LOMBARDI

This sounds harsh at first glance because society tells us to treat everyone the same. But reality is that doing so is one of the greatest causes of stress to dentists. To be successful, you have to consider that some people are ready to accept your recommendations while others are not. These two very different people require different amounts of time and energy.

Dave: *This runs counter to how I was raised: "treat everyone the same". But once I got beyond that head trash and defined who the top 20% percent of our patients were and how we would treat them as such AND the bottom 20% were and how should care for them differently...my practice growth became much more effortless.*

What does success mean to you?

Success is a never-ending process of repeatedly setting and achieving goals.

What is your morning routine (first 1–2 hrs of the day)?

Coffee, gets kids moving, get to work.

What is your biggest fear?

Don't really have one.

What is your goal-setting process?

I have an annual calendar on which I set out goals for the year. I created my own custom agenda/time-management tool in the form of a book that I use to track my to do list and next steps with ongoing projects.

What is the best investment you have made either inside your career or outside of dentistry?

Learning from experts. Mastermind participation. Free days and buffer days, taking time to think.

Looking back, what advice would you give yourself on the day of your dental school graduation?

Shoot first, ask questions later.

In your opinion, what separates the top 10% of dentists from the bottom 90%?

Executing on ideas. Being a fantastic communicator with a plan.

What keeps struggling dentists struggling?

Poor communication. Being indecisive.

If you had to narrow it down to a couple...what traits or skills do you think are most important in running an uncommonly successful practice?

1   Listening to patients to hear their frustrations and goals.

2   Effective marketing to identify people who want what you have.

3   Accepting that we are salespeople and making sure people get what they want.

What is a skill or procedure you've added since graduating from dental school that has had a major positive impact on your practice?

Cosmetic orthodontics/invisalign.

What is the best business advice you ever received?

It was a question: "Have you reached your quota of people you shouldn't be talking to or dealing with?" This led to me clearing my schedule (and much of life) of things I dislike and people who don't appreciate the value I offer.

What leadership advice would you give a dentist who has an ineffective culture in their practice?

Lead by example. Train staff relentlessly—there are training/learning moments every day.

What advice would you give a dentist that is struggling with case acceptance?

Practice communications. Study your patients. LISTEN to what patients want and give it to them. Stay "top of mind" with quality, consistent, relevant follow up.

What marketing advice would you give a dentist that is starting out in practice ownership?

Your marketing should change over time. Early on you need cashflow. Use offers to get people in the door. Provide red carpet service. Build credibility and social proof with reviews. Ask for referrals.

What do our dental patients most desire?

To be heard.

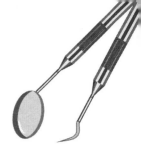

DR. BRUCE BAIRD

Granbury Dental Center,
Productive Dentist Academy,
Compassionate Finance

Justin: *I mentioned Dr. Blatchford as being one of the top 2 main influencers in my career. Well, Bruce is the other. If you haven't been to the Productive Dentist Academy yet, I suggest you get on it. Bill Blatchford suggested I go to PDA while we were doing our coaching, and I suggest it to all my clients. When it comes to producing dentistry, not many can top Bruce. He is a stud, and I'm forever grateful for the impact he has had on my life and career.*

Background

Dr. Baird graduated from the University of Texas Dental School in San Antonio in 1980. He spent 4 years as a dentist in the US Army from 1980–1984 and then opened up a private practice in Granbury, Texas where he still practices today.

Dr. Baird has lectured for the last 30 years throughout the world on dental implants, cosmetic dentistry, communication skills, business of dentistry, productivity, and the joys of being a dentist. He taught the senior class at Baylor Dental school on business and lectured at the Implant Preceptorship at the University of Texas Dental School in San Antonio.

He has been active in organized dentistry and has been selected as an Honored Fellow of the American Academy of Implant Dentistry, Diplomate of the International Congress of Implantology, and Fellow of the Academy of General Dentistry.

Dr. Baird has developed numerous dental techniques and methods of practice. In 2003, he founded the Productive Dentist Academy, which has grown over the last 14 years to include practice management, business, coaching, and an entire marketing department for dental practices. It began with 2 employees and today has over 40 team members. He also developed Comprehensive Finance in 2010. The company develops software and helps practices offer a new and innovative way of helping patients be able to have the care they need done while working within their budget. This company works with dental practices as well as numerous other professionals such as audiology, plastic surgery, ophthalmology, dermatology, and general physicians.

Please explain your style of practice (practice size, location, procedure mix, etc.)

I practice in Granbury, Texas. I've been here since 1984. My practice size is fairly large. I don't know what our total patient population is, but our average new patient drives over 50 miles, and I'll explain that later with marketing.

Right now, we have 23 employees with 3 full-time doctors. I've worked 2 days a week for the last 13 years. I still produce a significant amount of dentistry, actually more than I used to produce on 5 or 6 days. My procedure mix is dental implants, what I call Same-Day Smiles, which is, we use CEREC and CAD/CAM technology to be able to do 8 to 10 units in a single day. We start in the morning, and we seat into the afternoon.

I have a team member that does 90% of all of that for me; I just do the preparation, confirm the shape and size, and contacts, that type of thing, and then we go ahead and do it. I do lots of inlays and onlays using CEREC. My preference is to do materials such as an ENAMIC material on a posterior tooth, where the alternative would be composite resin. I just believe it's going to last longer. I also believe in giving patients the opportunity or the option to have something that's going to last 8 to 10 years or something that has a chance of lasting the rest of your life. They usually will choose the longer of those. So, they'll choose the onlays and inlays. That allows me to be very, very productive.

We pretty much keep everything in house. I'm not real fond of endodontics; my preference is to refer it among my partners, or refer out for that.

Do you have a favorite success quote or mantra?

One is, "Doing good while doing good." That's really our saying at Productive Dentists Academy. It's okay to be very successful and to make great money while you're helping more people.

The other quote is one from Tony Dungy's book, *Uncommon*. It's one of my favorite books, and it says, "Success is uncommon, therefore not to be enjoyed by the common man." Those are my two that I really look at more than anything.

Justin: Bruce turned me on to Tony's quote several years ago, and it has always stuck with me.

In regards to your dental career, what would you like your legacy to be, or how would you like to be remembered?

Somebody who had a lot of fun doing dentistry, who helped a lot of people become more productive, which in turn, allowed them more choices in their life to spend more time with their families, and spend more time with their kids.

Unfortunately, when I began, for my first 14 or 15 years, I was working 8 to 8 every day. It cost me dearly in family time and it took me a while to learn that there is a lot more important things to do rather than just make money, or try to be successful in dentistry.

Dentistry has become very successful for me. So, my legacy would be, you don't have to kill yourself. You can be very productive. You can make a fantastic living. More than 99.99% of the other people in the country, but also, it gives you the freedom to be able to have time to travel, time to play golf, time to spend with your kids, your grandkids, and everyone else.

Dave: *I have always admired Bruce's zest for life. We can all learn a lot from his pivot from focusing on working hard to focusing on working smart.*

What does success mean to you?

When I was 30 years old, it meant making a million dollars a year, or those types of things. As you get older, you start to realize you're only going to be on the planet for a short period of time, and my idea now would be I want to make a difference for people.

Success today to me, means pretty much where I'm at, which is, still working 2 days a week. I produce $2 million a year on 2 days a week. It allows me to have the income and revenue that I want. Also, having the extra time to be able to go travel, and to be able to go to all of the activities that my kids and grandkids have—that's what success means to me.

What is your morning routine (first 1-2 hrs of the day)?

I'm not one of those guys who gets up, and meditates, and does all of that stuff. I get up and say my prayers in the morning, but I tend to be more of an after-work guy. When I come home from work, that's when I work out. I usually spend 30 to 45 minutes working out in the evenings. I try to do that every day.

In the morning, I want to get to the office 15 to 20 minutes early, not to sit in our team meeting, because I put together an amazing team who know what their roles are. I think about my day. Where am I going to go first? What's the sequence of events that are going to happen? And then I trust my team to make that happen with me, and I give them that ability to be able to be a wonderful part of it.

What is your biggest fear?

Well, I'm 62 years old, and I don't really have a huge fear. I love my patients. I love my team that I work with. So, I'm very fortunate.

My biggest fear probably will be something happening to one of my grandkids or one of my children, or their family. That's the thing I think that concerns me.

Business-wise, I'm just not too worried about the business.

Please explain the most challenging time in your career and how you moved past it and thrived on the other side?

There is no question what that is. I was born the son of a Marine aviator, and everything was my way or the highway, which is black and white. It has to be done this way. Then I go to dental school. I learned, hey, it has to be done exactly this way or it's not going to work. I go into the service, it's very regimented. I get into private practice, and I start out in a small town of Granbury, of at the time, 3500 people. We were seeing mass numbers of new patients because we had a nuclear power plant right down the road. So, we were seeing 200–300 new patients a month, but I couldn't get them to say yes to treatment.

My team hated coming to work for me. I joked that almost everybody in town worked for me at one time or another. I was not a good boss. It had to be my way or the highway. I always use the term, "God has a sense of humor," because he gave me 4 daughters, and I would tell my girls, "All right girls, this is the way it's done." And they would start crying, and I would say, "Baby doll, that's not what I meant." And so, I had to learn to speak a different language.

I had to learn to empower people, and to become a leader instead of me putting my thumb down on people. I had to allow people to become successful, and that's helped me in every aspect of my life, from family to starting other businesses such as Compassionate Finance, and the Productive Dentist Academy. I've got wonderful teams that do an amazing, amazing job.

Dave: *I've talked to lots of highly successful dentists who have had a similar leadership epiphany at some point in their career that took them from a dictator to a developer of people. Many breakthroughs will occur when you make that shift.*

What is your goal-setting process?

I look at everything for 1, 3, and 5 years. I sit down and think this is the way I'd like to be, this is the kind of exercise I like to do, this is what I would like to see productivity-wise in our office, these are the goals that I would like to see happen with Compassionate Finance, with Productive Dentist Academy.

And then, we work backwards. And I follow—I get reports on a daily basis on where we're at. Monthly, I look at our reports and make sure that I'm reaching those goals.

I have a lot more personal goals now that have really nothing to do with dentistry, but you want to see certain things. I want to punch this or that on my bucket list. As you get older, you'll find that that's kind of what you start doing.

What is the best investment you have made either inside your career or outside of dentistry?

The best investment I've made is to understand that I didn't know everything when I got out of dental school, and even going into the service for 4 years.

I watched great dentists. People always rag on military dentists, but there are some phenomenal dentists there that have been wonderful practitioners in the military. I was able to learn a lot from them, but I realized I needed to learn more. Then when I got out—I've been a perpetual student for the last 38 years. I keep going to courses. I learn grafting. I learned connective tissue, I've learned different surgery techniques, and different materials, etc. What that has allowed me to do is be successful.

It has also allowed me to enjoy dentistry, even after doing it for 38 years. I love going to work. It has allowed me to be massively productive, to the tune of probably $3,000 an hour. Every day I work, I do $25,000 to $30,000 worth of dentistry. Now, you might say that's running around like a chicken with your head cut off, but the truth is, it really isn't. It's very easy to do that amount of dentistry, if you've learned the techniques, and you have a patient flow that allows you to be able to do that. So, that's the best investment...investing in myself.

I've invested in real estate. That's been great. I've learned a lot of lessons in investing in businesses. I've had some failures, but I also had some great successes. Being afraid to fail is not in my vocabulary.

Looking back, what advice would you give yourself on the day of your dental school graduation?

To be a perpetual student. Continue to learn, and do not quit.

Dave: *This is one of my favorite aspects of the profession. You've never quite mastered the clinical, business, or leadership aspect. There's always another level!*

In your opinion, what separates the top 10% of dentists from the bottom 90%?

They continually want to keep learning. They understand business, and that's something we don't get in dental school. I would go to business courses. I would learn communication skills. The top 10% really don't have much to do with their margins, or what kind of crown they do. It usually means they can communicate. Communication skills are absolutely the most important thing that you can learn, as long as you're doing wonderful dentistry. That's what keeps it fun.

What keeps struggling dentists struggling?

I think it's obvious. They think they know what they're doing, or they're afraid to fail. They'll keep doing the same thing, or they always feel like the world has been tough on them, their practice, their town, or their team. That's not it.

It's about becoming a leader. They keep struggling because they don't learn the things they need to. I had to learn to speak a different language. I had to learn to speak engineer when I was talking to engineers. I had to learn to do those things. It's not your patients or your team, it's usually because of us.

When I first started Productive Dentist Academy, I started with only the dentists, because most of the problems in a dental practice are because of the dentists. It really has nothing to do with the team.

You can have a team member that can be massively successful in one practice, go to another practice, and hate the office. It's not the person, it's the environment that we put them in.

What are the top 3 books every dental practice owner should read?

I've read some dental books, but most of the books I read are more for business.

1   *The Wow Factor* by Tom Peters is one of the originals. I began teaching 8 steps to wow back 30 years ago.

2   *Uncommon* by Tony Dungy

3   *Think and Grow Rich* by Napoleon Hill

If you had to narrow it down to a couple...what traits or skills do you think are most important in running an uncommonly successful practice?

Success is uncommon, therefore not to be enjoyed by the common man, in my opinion. The traits are communication skills and leadership; those are the two things—without communication skills and without leadership skills, it's very hard to be successful in practice.

I was massively unsuccessful the first 14 years, and then turned it around over the next 20 to be, what I consider, extremely successful by my measures. Having time, revenue, money, choices—those are the type of things I look for these days.

What is a skill or procedure you've added since graduating from dental school that has had a major positive impact on your practice?

Pretty much everything that I do has been added since graduating from dental school, from LANAP surgery, CAD/CAM; I mean, we didn't have microwaves when I graduated from dental school. So pretty much everything I do is something I didn't learn in dental school.

You don't learn a lot in dental school. We recently had a couple of young dentists that have been out for a year watch us do an over-the-shoulder program. They watched us for a day, and that evening we had cocktails and some dinner and one of them said, "I saw every procedure that we had to do as a requirement in dental school all done this morning by noon."

It's kind of funny, but it's the truth.

What is the best business advice you ever received?

Take care of your people. Take care of your team. People won't take care of your patients unless you're taking care of them. That's something from my perspective that is massively important.

Dave: I have a lot fewer "problems" on the days I show up to the practice to truly serve vs. the days I let my ego take over and start worrying about me. It dramatically affects the bottom line as well.

What advice would I give a dentist who has an ineffective culture in their practice?

I would say read, read, read. There are some great books on leadership out there. I would say one of the best that I've read is everything by Simon Sinek. Read all of his stuff, because it gets down to the gut reason why you're either a leader or not a leader. It's probably based on you, not so much on your team. If you have a bad team member, you'll know, but an ineffective culture has to do with the leader.

Dave: Accountability is also something where there's always another level. Climbing that ladder and pursuing the level where "everything is my fault" is incredibly powerful in practice and in life.

What advice would I give a dentist that's struggling with case acceptance?

I would say, learn the communication skills, because that's going to allow the case acceptance. At Productive Dentist Academy, we teach a specific way of doing risk factors, and working our way into a system so that patients say yes to treatment. All you have to do at that point is work out the financial arrangements.

I would read books on neurolinguistic programming, (Tony Robbins talks a lot about that) and books on communication skills.

What marketing advice would I give a dentist starting out in practice ownership?

Marketing doesn't happen overnight. Marketing is something that is an ongoing process. Marketing is everything you do. We recommend 8% of our budget. Meaning, if I collected $100,000, I have $8,000 to market. When the practice grew to $120K, my marketing budget went up, and so on.

A lot of people are too quick to sign up for PPOs that allow you a 30 to 40% discount, when the truth is, if you plan for those expenditures to start with, that I'm going to have a marketing budget—and whatever it is, you continue to market using that budget.

I have a story of two dentists, both in the same town. One had been practicing for years and had even written books on practice management of the PPO-type practice. I asked him, "Have you ever tried marketing?" He said, "Oh yeah, I've marketed everywhere. It just doesn't work. Everyone in my town is on some type of plan, so I have to do that." I said, "Okay."

The next seminar, I had somebody else from the same town. A young female dentist, who'd been out of school 3 years. She took no plans at all, and actually was seeing lots of new patients that were all fee-for-service patients. So, they're not discounting their fees up front, and they're actually using money to market towards the type of people that needed the work.

That's what I would say for somebody starting out. Start out with a plan.

Justin: *I've used Bruce's example countless times when it comes to marketing. I've often told others...the most productive dentist I know spends the most on marketing of any dentist I know. That's not to take away from Bruce in any way. You could give his marketing budget to someone else and most are not going to be able to replicate what he does. However, I know not shying away on his marketing, even once he was very successful, has continued to fuel his fire, and allowed him to consistently produce at a very high level year after year.*

What do our dental patients most desire?

They want stuff done quickly, efficiently, and they don't want to be hurt. That is why we do a lot of same-day dentistry. When they come in, my goal is to get them treated. They want to be treated compassionately. They want to feel like when they leave, they're leaving their friends.

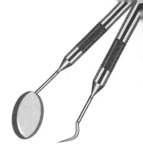

DR. APRIL ZIEGELE

Ziegele Smile Studio

Justin: *I actually had the privilege of spending the day in April's office several years ago, while in Seattle for a course at the Kois Center. I met April at a seminar when I was going through coaching with Bill Blatchford, but it didn't take long for me to recognize the way in which her team carried themselves and to see there was something "different" there. April and her team are anything but common.*

I was a bit reluctant to call her out of the blue and ask to come visit her and her office. Needless to say, she was very welcoming, and spending the day observing how she runs her practices, and how April and her team treat their "guests" was worth the price of admission many times over.

I'm glad I made that call, because the few pearls I picked up that day forever changed how I ran my practices from that day forward. Thanks, April!

Background

I received my doctorate in dentistry from Loma Linda University School of Dentistry and graduated at the top of my class in 1997. I have trained at the world-renowned Las Vegas Institute for Advanced Dental Studies and have been featured in a book by Dr. Bill Blatchford about the top 23 dentists in North America, called *Playing Your 'A' Game.*

I am active in the American Academy of Cosmetic Dentistry, the American Dental Association, the American Academy of Facial Esthetics, the Las Vegas Institute for Advanced Dental Studies, the International Association of Esthetic Dentistry, the American Academy of Implant Dentistry, the Academy of Comprehensive Esthetics, and the California Implant Institute.

Personally, my husband Jon and I have been married for almost 22 years, and have 2 children. Christopher, 18, is heading to college this year and wants to be an oral surgeon. Lauren, 16, is still in high school and will likely do something where she can utilize her artistic skills. As a family, we love the ocean, and all things water. My preference for a vacation will always involve a beach. My kids and I are all certified lifeguards and love swimming any chance we get. We have 3 small dogs at home, one of which is our office Therapy Dog, Moose. Our patients adore Moose and he gives so much comfort and love to everyone!

As an office team, we find at least one day each year to give back. That's very important to me. This year, my son and I went to the Philippines for a 2-week mission trip where we extracted teeth all day long, every single day.

Please explain your style of practice (practice size, location, procedure mix, etc.)

We practice in a small town in Southwest Washington state. We always tell people we're from Seattle, because nobody knows where Sumner is, even if they're FROM Washington state! But really, we're about 45 miles outside of Seattle. It's a small enough area that where I live we have cows in our subdivision. We run into patients all the time at grocery stores, and I love that.

We do a pretty big mix of everything in the practice, but I don't place implants any longer. I did for a while, but after taking the full practicon on implants, and placing about 20 of them, I discovered that I really, really hated surgery. So I quit doing it. Life is simply too short to do the things that you hate.

Do you have a favorite success quote or mantra?

> *"If you set your goals ridiculously high and it's a*
> *failure, you will fail above everyone else's success."*

> —JAMES CAMERON

In regards to your dental career, what would you like your legacy to be, or how would you like to be remembered?

I'd like to be remembered as someone who lived with integrity, who used every opportunity to lift up others around me, who found ways to give to others.

What does success mean to you?

Success is being happy with who I am at the end of the day. To look back at the day, and think, "I did enough."

What is your morning routine (first 1–2 hrs of the day)?

Get up, take the dogs outside with a cup of tea and the book I'm currently reading. Read while outside with them for 20 minutes, then spend another 10 minutes planning out my day. Shower, get ready, listen to Christian music, grab a protein bar, get in the car, listen to an audiobook on my way to work. I am always at work about an hour before everyone else, and I really like that quiet time to get things ready, get anything done that I need to do, just get prepared.

What is your biggest fear?

Not being enough.

Please explain the most challenging time in your career and how you moved past it and thrived on the other side?

I went through a lawsuit with a former employee who I had thought of also as a close friend. It was jarring, life altering, and devastating. I kind of crawled into myself for about a year, just utterly gutted by the entire thing. I couldn't understand why this had happened, but then I began to climb out of it with the help of a great family support system and team.

What is your goal-setting process?

I look out 10 years, and then move backward to 6 months.

What is the best investment you have made either inside your career or outside of dentistry?

Hiring a dental coach.

Looking back, what advice would you give yourself on the day of your dental school graduation?

Make some dental friends. It's a very lonely career sometimes.

Dave: *I was very independent in my early career. I thought every problem had its solution in hard work. I can tell you that all of my career breakthroughs in the last 5 years has come from developing trusting friendships with colleagues around the country that have similar mindsets. The support and synergy of ideas is powerful beyond measure.*

In your opinion, what separates the top 10% of dentists from the bottom 90%?

A very, very tiny bit. Just doing that one more thing, is the difference. One more class to have a tiny bit more knowledge, one more step taken consistently, the consistent post-op calls in the evening.

Justin: I loved this answer when I read it. I'm a big believer in nailing the simple things day after day. The most successful dentists I know consistently execute on the handful of simple things we all encounter each day in our offices, as opposed to constantly trying to master every new idea that crosses their path.

What keeps struggling dentists struggling?

I believe it's because they're embarrassed and don't reach out for help. For starters, we're trained to pick each other to death, so reaching out is a bit terrifying.

What are the top 3 books every dental practice owner should read?

Good to Great by Jim Collins
The Year of Yes by Shonda Rhimes
The Fred Factor (and *Fred Factor 2.0*) by Mark Sanborn

If you had to narrow it down to a couple...what traits or skills do you think are most important in running an uncommonly successful practice?

Paying attention to the numbers every single month. Treating your team outrageously well—they pass that along to the patients.

What is a skill or procedure you've added since graduating from dental school that has had a major positive impact on your practice?

Full arch or full mouth restorative procedures while maintaining a bite. LVI had a great impact on me. I never understood CR and it was really uncomfortable to me to be in that position. They gave me an option that made sense, and in that way I felt able to restore beauty with function.

What is the best business advice you ever received?

Treat employees the way you want your patients to be treated.

What leadership advice would you give a dentist who has an ineffective culture in their practice?

It starts with you. What are you projecting when you walk into your office? The attitude and culture starts with the person you see in the mirror. If you want an actual change, take a hard look at what you are doing and change yourself.

Dave: Agreed! Accountability is hard. But, if you can come to terms with the idea that you are the problem...then, you have control over the solution.

What advice would you give a dentist that is struggling with case acceptance?

If you feel desperate, the patients can certainly feel it. But when you are coming from a place of abundance, they want what you have. If you are trying to "educate them into acceptance," it will never work. If knowledge were all it took, you'd never see a dentist with a cavity, or a physician that's overweight.

What marketing advice would you give a dentist that is starting out in practice ownership?

Commit to a percentage at the beginning and never vary from it. When times are tough, it's especially important to market yourself.

What do our dental patients most desire?

They want to look good and feel good.

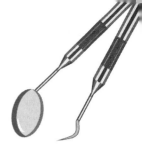

DR. ALAN MEAD

Mead Family Dental,
Dental Hacks, and
The Alan Mead Experience Podcasts

Justin: *I know Dave and Alan are friends as well, but I was the one who got the chance to discuss this project with Alan. I think Alan would be ok with me telling this, but he was a bit reluctant to do the interview. I never got the impression that he didn't want to help, but Alan is self-admittedly not the multi-million dollar practice "gunner". I actually love that about Alan.*

On the flip side, where he stands out to me in regards to "greatness of achievement" is in his passion for podcasting. Not only producing 2 top-rated dental podcasts, but also being willing to help others on their journey into the world of podcasting. He stays true to himself, which in our mind is a hallmark of any Titan.

Background

I was born and raised in Midland, MI...the same town where I now live. My dad was a dentist, and I grew up in a dental office and dental culture. I mowed the office lawn as soon as I was 12 or so (I was horrible...well known for destroying in-ground sprinkler heads). We used to go to Chicago in February all the time. I never realized that it was for midwinter. I just knew that my mom took us to Shedd's Aquarium, the museum, and shopping on the Miracle Mile. I graduated from the University of Minnesota School of Dentistry in 1997.

In 1998, I bought a practice in Saginaw, MI (the same practice I'm in now), but left dental practice for 4 1/2 months to go into drug treatment in 2002. I've been clean and sober ever since. I began speaking about addiction in 2008. I also used to speak about social media as well as medical marijuana. In 2014, I started the *Dental Hacks* podcast with Dr. Jason Lipscomb. In 2016, we started the *Dental Hacks Nation* Facebook group, which has grown to over 20,000 people and in 2017, I started *The Alan Mead Experience* podcast. I also helped start *The Voices of Dentistry* meeting in 2016. The VoD is a "dental podcast"–centered meeting and like nothing the dental industry has ever seen!

Please explain your style of practice (practice size, location, procedure mix, etc.)

By most standards, I have a tiny practice. It's bread and butter. Mostly restorative with a little surgery and endo on occasion.

Do you have a favorite success quote or mantra?

No. I kind of hate that stuff, actually.

In regards to your dental career, what would you like your legacy to be, or how would you like to be remembered?

I'd like to be remembered as a good dentist by my patients and a guy that helped bring dental podcasting onto the scene by dentists and dental people.

What does success mean to you?

Doing as much or as little as I want to do and being financially stable enough to do it. Spending time with my family and having as much time to create stuff as I want.

What is your morning routine (first 1–2 hrs of the day)?

Usually it involves a cup of coffee and then feeding horses.

What is your biggest fear?

I can't really think of a "biggest fear." I'm not fearless at all. It's just that the things that cause anxiety and fear in me are silly, day-to-day things. My biggest fear last week probably doesn't even show up on the radar this week.

Please explain the most challenging time in your career and how you moved past it and thrived on the other side?

The first few years of owning my own practice were the most challenging. Mostly because I was an active drug addict. But not only that, I was unprepared to be an owner. In the late 90s, the resources for owners were harder to come by. The internet, podcasts, and social media have really changed that.

Dave: *One of the main reasons I started the Relentless Dentist podcast was that I thought dentistry needed more authenticity, more willingness to be upfront about the struggles. Of all the guests I've had on the show, few have been as vulnerable as Alan was. He recognizes that one of the best ways to help our colleagues is by creating an understanding that some of us have deep and dark challenges during our career. With persistence and support, we can find success and fulfillment on the other side of it.*

What is your goal-setting process?

I'd love to tell you that I have one, but I really don't. Interestingly, the changes that I choose to make in my life and my office are the ideas that tend to recur in my daily life. For instance...I was obsessed with dental microscopes for years. I would continue to talk myself out of getting one, but the idea would continue to crop up. I don't know if that qualifies as goal setting, but it's worked for me.

What is the best investment you have made either inside your career or outside of dentistry?

Starting a podcast. I know that doesn't seem like "an investment", but it totally is. I invested a few thousand in equipment, but I really invested a lot of my time into learning how to do it and just doing it. The payoff has been that I get to talk with all these amazing people in dentistry and create a lot of cool stuff.

Looking back, what advice would you give yourself on the day of your dental school graduation?

Stop drinking. Don't take mood-altering chemicals. Some people can do this, but you can't. That said...my journey may well have made me the person I am. Also...I totally wouldn't have listened.

What keeps struggling dentists struggling?

I'm going to say some self-reflection and maybe a little meditation can help anyone who is struggling.

What are the top 3 books every dental practice owner should read?

Small is the New Big by Seth Godin
The Dip by Seth Godin
Stoicism: A Stoic Approach to Modern Life by Tom Miles

If you had to narrow it down to a couple...what traits or skills do you think are most important in running an uncommonly successful practice?

Self-reflection, skepticism, and communication.

What is a skill or procedure you've added since graduating from dental school that has had a major positive impact on your practice?

Using a dental operating microscope. My diagnostic abilities are so much better with a scope than without. The precision of the dentistry I can deliver is also much greater. The scope is useful across so many different parts of dentistry and you just can't do documentation any better.

What is the best business advice you ever received?

Spend less than you earn.

What leadership advice would you give a dentist who has an ineffective culture in their practice?

The only person that will be there until the place is closed or sold is you. So build the practice to work for you.

What advice would you give a dentist that is struggling with case acceptance?

Your obligation to the patient is to show them their condition. Do that well. Answer their questions. Suggest treatment that you're sure will make their condition better. Then let them choose. Some will, some won't. That's OK. I'd much rather work on a patient that chose my treatment from understanding their condition than one who felt like I'd talked them into it.

What marketing advice would you give a dentist that is starting out in practice ownership?

Start a blog. It's super cheap (almost free except for the time you put into it) and Google loves it. Use photos and stories to let people know why you're different.

What do our dental patients most desire?

Understanding and being met where they are.

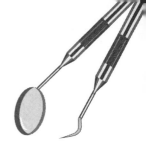

DR. BRADY FRANK

Premier Care Dental, Speaker,
Author of Transition Time

Background

After a potentially career-ending wrist injury as a junior in dental school, Dr. Brady Frank realized that he could not rely solely on the clinical practice of dentistry for his income.

Beginning in 1999, Brady began researching top entrepreneurs and differing streams of income both within dentistry and outside dentistry. One such favored model to building non-clinical income is the multi-location, multi-doctor group. Dr. Frank closed on one practice and dental building immediately upon graduation, another practice 6 months later, and within 7 years, had purchased 12 practices and employed 28 associates.

To this day, Dr. Frank continues to co-own private dental group practices (DDSOs) and build associated multiple streams of income and vertical companies. His passion, however, is teaching other dentists his techniques so that dentistry becomes a CHOICE rather than a NECESSITY from a financial standpoint.

Please explain your style of practice
(practice size, location, procedure mix, etc.)

My favorite practice opportunity is what I call the Value-Added Practice Acquisition or Entrepreneurial Satellite Practice, or ESP. This implies the practice you're purchasing will achieve some sort of investment objectives. I coined this term more than a decade ago when referring to the 12 practices I purchased within 7 years after I graduated from dental school.

In these situations, the investment return is often very profitable, but you do lose the practice's cash flow. That means you forfeit all the growth momentum, but by using the models I've illustrated throughout my book, you can have the proverbial cake and eat it too. That's because ESPs with a continual exit strategy provide a return of capital, a cash investment return, monthly cash flow, elimination of debt, and future equity growth.

After a full day of lecturing on this topic, a dentist approached me and regretfully said, "I wish I would have attended this lecture a year ago, prior to selling my $5 million practice." He then went on to explain that after taxes were paid on the sale price and net funds invested, he found himself living off 90% less monthly income than before he sold the practice. Ouch. That's a pretty significant drop that could have been avoided if he had followed this model.

You probably know there are three main parts to any implant procedure—the fixture itself, the abutment, and finally the prosthetic loading the abutment. There are also three main aspects with every practice acquisition: finding, funding, and farming. Finding involves locating the opportunity, funding involves the financial structure of the transaction from cash to seller-financing to third-party financing, and farming involves the transitional management and increase of the acquired practice. Finding an outstanding acquisition value and achieving high investment returns are my favorite practice opportunities!

Do you have a favorite success quote or mantra?

"If you help enough people get what THEY want,
you will eventually get what you want."

—ZIG ZIGLAR

In regards to your dental career, what would you like your legacy to be, or how would you like to be remembered?

I would like to be known as someone who helped colleagues with tools, techniques, and opportunities allowing them to reach their maximum potential personally, professionally, and financially.

What does success mean to you?

Success to me is having total freedom to pursue that which is most important. Total freedom relates to financial freedom, personal freedom, and time freedom. This definition of success leads to influence, which leads to significance.

Dave: *I appreciate this comprehensive look at freedom. I see too many dentists pursuing the financial goals that will leave them without time or geographic freedom.*

What is your morning routine (first 1–2 hrs of the day)?

I like to write in the early mornings before my wife and 3 boys are out of bed. Oftentimes I will hike in the pre-dawn darkness as I mentally map out more complex components to my DDSO clients' growth and acquisition plans.

What is your biggest fear?

My biggest fear is that I would quit one of my main purposes, serving others, so that I can arrive safely at death.

Justin: I like Brady's phrasing here. Of course we need to utilize wisdom, but how often do we avoid perceived risks in life to arrive more "safely at death"?

Please explain the most challenging time in your career and how you moved past it and thrived on the other side?

I have encountered multiple mountains in my career where the future seemed uncertain, wrought with potentially insurmountable risk, and with very little clarity for the path moving forward. Thankfully, in my weakness I have found strength being a person of faith. Strength to strategize, be creative, take action, and make the moves needed to scale the mountain and find myself in a better place having gone through that adversity. The business of dentistry is all about solving problems. The dentist that solves the most problems, with the best solutions and most viable time-tested models, finds success.

Dave: Too often in my career was I naive enough to wish the problems in my practice would go away. When I shifted my paradigm to accepting and anticipating the problems (not just clinical, but the business, staffing, and upset patient problems), my enjoyment increased dramatically. I had spent way too much time "arguing with reality" and that causes great stress.

What is your goal-setting process?

As Stephen Covey stated in *The 7 Habits of Highly Effective People,* "Begin with the end in mind." Before I set any goal, I first envision the outcome of achieving that goal. I believe many would choose entirely different goals if they truly understood the outcome in the achievement of certain goals.

There is also a process I like to employ called "goal stacking". By beginning with the end in mind, it is likely that several of your goals hinge on the successful completion of just one of those goals. So by taking down "the Golden Goal", you automatically achieve 3–5 other goals. The goals were stacked together. You may liken it to the one big domino, that once achieved, easily knocks down all the others. The key is to understand which one is the big domino, the Golden Goal!

What is the best investment you have made either inside your career or outside of dentistry?

I would have to say my investment in continuing education related to multiple streams of income OUTSIDE of dentistry that I have been able to apply within DDSO concepts INSIDE dentistry.

Looking back, what advice would you give yourself on the day of your dental school graduation?

When you hit a roadblock or obstacle or find failure, fear not! For it is the process of pushing through those adversities that true, lasting success is found.

Dave: *This is a perfect opportunity for me to encourage you to read one of my favorite books of all time. It's on this very subject of turning obstacles into opportunities. It's* The Obstacle is the Way *by Ryan Holiday.*

In your opinion, what separates the top 10% of dentists from the bottom 90%?

Their inner circle combined with their inner drive toward achievement.

What keeps struggling dentists struggling?

Struggling dentists continue to struggle for two reasons. Firstly, due to lack of access to specialized knowledge needed to overcome. Secondarily, due to refusing to accept responsibility, which allows one to continually blame external circumstances rather than themselves.

If you had to narrow it down to a couple...what traits or skills do you think are most important in running an uncommonly successful practice?

Acquiring the right information and taking massive action.

What is a skill or procedure you've added since graduating from dental school that has had a major positive impact on your practice?

How to acquire value-added practices with little to no money down and convert positive equity growth into debt-reduction and tax-advantaged wealth acceleration.

What is the best business advice you ever received?

Understand WHY you are growing a business prior to growing that business. There are many destitute folks who have brilliant business success stories.

What leadership advice would you give a dentist who has an ineffective culture in their practice?

Learn how to be a Servant Leader. Serve your staff and patients. Take the garbage to the dumpster.

What advice would you give a dentist that is struggling with case acceptance?

Start off telling the patient your philosophy: The best dentistry is no dentistry. The next best thing is dentistry that prevents more major dentistry (like a crown to help prevent a root canal). The walls go down!

What marketing advice would you give a dentist that is starting out in practice ownership?

Understand that marketing is the best pre-tax investment.

What do our dental patients most desire?

To be understood. We must seek first to understand BEFORE we are understood.

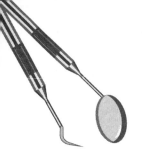

DR. DAVID PHELPS

Freedom Founders

Justin: *I first came across David a few years ago, and thought, "How have I not found him sooner?" David and I have many similar beliefs about life, and I enjoy any chance we get to talk. In 2017, I was fortunate enough to attend one of his events with Freedom Founders. I had the chance to meet some incredible forward-thinking doctors, and overall it was a great experience. Even though David is a dentist by trade, he has achieved freedom and wealth using real estate, a topic near and dear to my heart.*

I think his approach to life and wealth creation differs from most dentists. Not that one is right and one is wrong, but we think you'll enjoy a different perspective than that of many wet-fingered dentists.

Background

I started investing in real estate my first year in dental school, so I tell people I was really a real estate investor before I became a dentist. Then I came out of dental school and sold that first property. I took about a $25,000 capital gain profit, and rolled that into the next properties, and just continued to practice dentistry, and become the best dentist I could during the day.

I took a lot of CE, but I also was involved, probably as much, in real estate and doing a lot of courses there, and finding the right mentors in real estate.

Sometimes as type-A people, we put our families on the back burner because we think, someday, when I get all of this other stuff right, when I get it where I want it, then I'll start living. For too many people, you never get there. There has to be a balance, as hard as it is to get there.

I both ran the practice and built-up real estate. Then my daughter got leukemia at age two-and-a-half; that was back in the early 90s. She survived that, but then she had epileptic seizures from age 8 to 12, which was, again, a huge emotional and physical battle.

It was detrimental to our family, insomuch as I lost the marriage in 1998. Jenna was 6. Then she had to have a liver transplant at age 12. A lot of things blew up early in my life that I had no idea would be challenges. I thought, like a lot of us, if you do the work—if you're smart enough to get the grades, and get through school, then we can make it.

I realized more and more with age, wisdom, and maturity, to expect to have things not go your way. Not things that you did because of your own recklessness or negligence, but things will just happen that you have no control over many times, and you have to expect those things to happen somewhere.

You just have to have a mindset. You know what? I can work really hard and do the right things in life, but at some point, something is going to happen that I don't expect. Are you resilient enough—are you prepared enough with the mindset to deal with that?

Anyway, I decided in 2004, when Jenna had the liver transplant, that basically I was done being a scheduled, 4-day-a-week dentist running a practice. I had enough real estate to let it go, but I needed permission.

A big thing that I talk to people about is you've got to have a why to get out of your comfort zone. You've got to have a why to push you beyond your safety net. Because if you're getting up on Monday morning to go into the office, and Sunday night you dread it, trust me, you're not living the life you need to be living.

I had that feeling. I had Sunday nights where it's like, "God dang, I've got to go to the office tomorrow?" I'd rather be doing real estate. Finally, with Jenna's illness and her ultimate liver transplant, I had my own personal permission, without apologizing to anybody, including myself, to say, "I'm done".

I'm going to go do a different life. Right then and there, it was based on my daughter. Nothing else. I'll get my financial lifestyle nut down to whatever it needs to be, to let the real estate produce it so I can spend time with her, because I was sick and tired of going back and forth from the office, feeling that pull back, and then leaving her in the hospital, you know, wherever she was at this time. She can be gone tomorrow, and here I am running back to the office to treat more patients.

After I left the practice, it was like, wow. I mean, I'm really, really free of that darn ball and chain. I really can start figuring out what's next and that's what led to the creation of Freedom Founders.

Do you have a favorite success quote or mantra?

There is no such day in the week called "Someday". I think too many people put off living purposeful, meaningful, significant lives because they think that when they get certain things done in life, that "Someday" will arrive, and that "Someday" is when they will start living.

The problem for most people is "Someday" never arrives.

In regards to your career or in Freedom Founders, what would you like your legacy to be or, how would you like to be remembered?

I'd like to be remembered as someone who is respected in the communities in which I revolve. A person of high integrity, who cared for his patients and staff when I was in practice. Foremost, that I cared about the people that I have the privilege, or the honor, to touch or influence.

I take that with a huge responsibility. First and foremost, to be 100% authentic, and speak the truth, and only the truth, about what I've learned in life.

Dave: Dr. Phelps was one of my first podcast guests. We became fast friends due to our similar life philosophies. I admired his authenticity from day one. He invited me to one of the first Freedom Founders meetings in Dallas. It was inspiring to see him in action, providing an alternative roadmap to dentists who were feeling like they were a prisoner in their own practice.

What does success mean to you?

I think success is a word, that is used a lot today, and is certainly going to be different for everybody. For me, I think you've got to combine whatever your definition of success is, and for some people that's a financial number, it's a monetary number, or it may be a lifestyle number.

But I think until you add significance to success, that you really don't have the full meaning of what success means. Success should be— that you have the freedom, the option, so that you're empowered so that you can give to other people. I think that's the true meaning of success. That's what mine would be.

What is your morning routine? The first 1–2 hours of the day?

Typically, I'll start by doing some reading. I've always got stacks of books by the bedside, or on the Kindle. I'll start by reading; naturally that gets my mind thinking—just gets my head working for that day a little bit. Then pretty quickly, I jump in and take care of any messaging that I need to get to my team.

A lot of people say, "Well, don't get into your email, your inbox, early." I take the other approach. I get in early, get stuff out, so I'm not the bottleneck. I'm not the constraint. I get some people working on projects. I get that stuff off my plate early. That's typically how I get started, the first couple of hours.

What is your biggest fear?

That time will run out, and I won't be able to fully impact as many people as I would like to impact or influence.

Please explain the most challenging time in your career and how you moved past it to thrive on the other side?

That's the failed practice sale, back in 2006 after I made the decision to sell. I sold to a very charismatic, very clinically gifted young doctor, and his credit was not quite what it needed to be to buy me out with bank financing, so I carried the paper, fully believing that within a year, he would have the financial track record as the owner of the business to refinance me out.

Unfortunately, there were some character issues that caused that transaction to fail, and I had to take the practice back, through some legal contortions, which is never good for anybody.

It certainly wasn't good for the practice, the staff, or the patients. But I did get it back. I made a commitment to myself, as I knew I was going to get the practice back, that I was not going to go back in and be the doctor again in providing the services.

I was not going to go back into that. I had to change the way I thought about that practice. I took what I learned over the years about marketing, and brought in three associates. Three different associates over a period of about 5 months to expand the hours of the practice, and to have not just 1, or 2, but to have this time 3 people from whom I would have the opportunity to choose from, who can be the buyer of the practice. Three years later, that consummated.

What I learned was, is that dentistry, the practice of dentistry, actually can be run as a real business. We know, certainly, corporations are doing that right and left today, but what about the smaller practice?

I learned I didn't have to be the primary producer at the practice. That it could be run well with—in this case, associates, associates that had an opportunity to move into ownership, and I think there is a difference there, versus an associate who has no current opportunity to buy in. They have a different mindset.

Big lessons are, it doesn't all have to be on you, even though in our own heads, many times we think that we have to do it all. That no one else could do it as well as we can. That's not a good mindset, and that will hold people back from fulfilling their real dreams and real passion in life, if they think that way.

What is your goal setting process currently?

When I have a goal or an outcome that I wish to reach, whatever that might be—that might be in certain investments, that might be cash flow, that might be time freedom, that might be something else for Freedom Founders—whatever it is, I will define as precisely or specifically as I can, what that goal looks like when it's complete.

I think that's the key, is you've got to be very precise. If that's with numbers, be precise. If it's with a lifestyle, if it's the way your company looks, or whatever it is, you've got to be precise. You've got to be able to envision it and get those details down, so you can really, really see it.

Once you've got the clarity of what that outcome or that goal is going to look like when you reach it, then you've got to reverse engineer. I know what the destination looks like, now, where am I starting from? Then you've got to determine, what's the gap in between? Start to find the gap, and how do you start breaking the gap down into steps? What are the steps I've got to take to start reaching it?

I think a lot of people have goals, but they're fuzzy. They don't put enough specifics in them. They don't put time deadlines or milestones into them. You've got to have those in place. You may not hit all of those exactly when you need to, but at least you've got a way to measure progress on a regular basis.

What is the best investment you've made, either inside your career, or outside of dentistry?

For me, it's relationships. I always call it what it is; it's relationship capital. It's other people. It's other people who could be your mentors, or other people who are like-minded.

Your circle of influence. The people you surround yourself with. Jim Rohn said it best: "You become the average of the five people you most associate with." I think that's really true; you've got to really consider who you spend time with outside your family.

Who do you spend time with? Who do you talk to? Who do you brainstorm with? If they're not the right people, then you're going to stay at a certain point in your life. Your thinking is not going to expand.

We all have some kind of defined limits from our environment, right? I think the goal for all of us is to be around people who help us expand, and push back, and make us get a little uncomfortable where we are. I think it's a good thing to be uncomfortable, and to be looking at—what can I be changing for the better?

It all comes from people, in my opinion.

Looking back, what advice would you give yourself on the day of dental school graduation?

Another great question. I would say finding the absolute best mentor. Ideally you want to gain a connection, a relationship, with that mentor. How do you do that? Well, you do that by finding some way to serve usually first.

School is just that first baby step, it's that first right of passage that lets you take the next step, but so much more is beyond that. Finding that right person and getting that mentorship, I think, for the first couple of years, is really important.

Dave: *David brings up a great point about serving or adding value. You can expect most people who you'd like to have as a mentor are extremely busy. How can you make it a win-win relationship for them?*

In your opinion, what separates the top 10% of dentists from the bottom 90%?

It's certainly not clinical skills, and too many people think that that's where it's at. I would say it's business acumen, combined with communication and leadership skills. That's where it is in any business, and continued education of your clinical skills, your patient diagnosis, treatment planning, pride of service is also important.

If you want to be successful today, you've got to have business acumen, communication, relationship skills, all of the stuff that we were never taught in school. Those all can be learned, but it takes dedication to go there.

Most people think "Well, nope. I just need to be a better dentist." They focus all on that, and there again, there is a ceiling on that, because if you can't run a business, if you can't market, if you can't communicate well, you don't have leadership; you're going to hit a ceiling.

What keeps struggling dentists struggling?

I think it's fear of change. We get to a point in life where success is actually a trap. Success as in I'm paying the bills, I'm providing for my family, I'm in good shape. That success is a trap, and so it's fear of change. It's fear of upsetting that level of comfort for something that could be a lot better.

I think it's being closed-minded. Fear of change, inability to take action, not knowing what they don't know, not being coachable or open to mentoring, I think are the biggest points of struggle for most people who aren't where they want to be.

What are the top 3 books every dental practice owner should read?

The E-Myth by Michael Gerber.
Leaders Eat Last by Simon Sinek; that's a great leadership book.
Good to Great by Jim Collins.

At Freedom Founders—I did not do this with my dental practice, but I would do it today—we do a book study. We choose books like these that talk about culture, leadership, systems, processes, and people in the right seats, and we do a book study where we we talk about them once a week. A lot of good comes from that. I love books, and those would be probably the top 3 that I would suggest.

If you had to narrow it down to a couple, what traits or skills do you think are most important in running an uncommonly successful practice?

I think it would be marketing and communication skills. It goes a little bit hand in hand. Marketing is communication. Also, learning how to market to the ideal patient niche that you're looking for, and being able to do that effectively. Then having personal communication skills, certainly communication skills throughout your whole team and practice.

What is a skill or a procedure you added since graduation that has had a major positive impact on your practice?

I would say leadership, and learning to be a much better leader. I don't think I had much in the way of leadership skills. I probably tried to be a good leader, but I didn't know how to be a good leader. I think being a good leader, both for your own family and for your practice, and being a good leader in the community, is one of the greatest skill sets that I've added over the years of my life.

That's probably allowed me to go further, and live a better life, and live a life of significance much more than when I didn't focus on having better leadership skills.

What is the best business advice you have received?

I'll go back to that relationship capital. Surrounding yourself with people that are wiser and more experienced than you are. People that have already gone down a path that you seek to also reach, and just being around them. Do what you have to do.

Serve them, pay to play, but whatever it is, make sure that you are among people that have already gone down a path that you wish to go down.

What leadership advice would you give a dentist who has an ineffective culture in their practice?

Get help. Again, this is where you've got to reach out and just realize that you don't know everything. You may be a great dentist, but you're not a great leader at this point. You have not figured out how to hire correctly and build that culture.

Get a mentor. Get a coach. Learn how to be a better leader. I think that's one of the biggest things that's missing in most businesses, whether dentistry or not, is that the business owner just doesn't know what he doesn't know.

Being a leader is often not innate; we just do what we've seen other people do, and usually it's not very effective.

What advice would you give a dentist that is struggling with case acceptance?

I think, first and foremost, I would look to see what the self-confidence of that dentist is.

In other words, their ability to confidently provide a wider spectrum of treatment, is not there. If that's the case, then certainly, that's going to hurt case acceptance, right? They're not going to diagnose it, or if the hygienist diagnoses it, they're going to push back because they're a little afraid of doing the implant. They're afraid of doing the root canal. They're afraid of whatever.

Then the second part, we're going back to your communication skills. Within the whole office, not just the dentist, to convert a patient's treatment needs into acceptance. Self-confidence and communication would be the keys there that I think need to be focused on.

What do our dental patients most desire? I'd also be curious on your perspective: what do dentists you work with most desire?

I think everybody wants truthful communication. They want people who are going to, in this case, consult on dental oral health needs, or advise or consult like we do at Freedom Founders on wealth building through real estate; people want the truth.

They don't want to be sold something that's not right for them. They want somebody who is in a position to offer them really the best options for that person, and not offering options because that person or that company needs to make a certain dollar amount off of this case or this particular perspective member.

Truthful communication that has the best interests of the person in mind, I think is what people really want today.

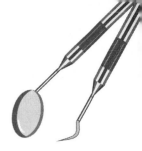

DR. PETER DAWSON

The Dawson Academy

Dave: *I had the honor of doing this interview in person. I don't use the term honor lightly. Dr. Dawson was the guest of honor at the Christian Medical and Dental Associations' Dawson Retreat that happened to be at a resort in the same town where I practice.*

We had tried to do the interview via phone, but Dr. Dawson insisted that we do it in person. He was generous with his time and so thoughtful in his answers. Having that one-on-one time with him was one of the highlights of my career. As you'll see in his answers that follow, his wisdom isn't limited to the clinical principles that he's famous for.

Background

Peter E. Dawson, D.D.S. is considered to be one of the most influential clinicians and teachers in the history of dentistry. He authored the best-selling dental text, *Evaluation, Diagnosis and Treatment of Occlusal Problems*, which is published in 13 languages. His latest book is entitled *Functional Occlusion: From TMJ to Smile Design*. He is the founder of the "Concept of Complete Dentistry Seminar Series (SM)" as well as The Dawson Academy.

In addition to numerous awards and special recognitions, Dr. Dawson is the past president and life member of the American Equilibration Society and a past president of the American Academy of Restorative Dentistry and the American Academy of Esthetic Dentistry.

Please tell us a little about the Dawson Academy

At The Dawson Academy, we have the opportunity to get to know dentists from all over the world. We've had over 50,000 dentists that have come through. We always try to ask a lot of questions regarding what they know. We have come to the very strong conclusion, that dentists do not know what they do not know. When they don't know what they don't know, they don't know they need to know it.

Number one on the list of things that dentists are not being taught in dental schools, which is the basis for predictability of everything they do, is occlusion. If you don't understand occlusion to a degree that you can be predictable in diagnosing the problem of occlusion, and how to treat problems of occlusion, then you're going to have a frustrating practice, because you'll have no predictability.

The thing that frustrates us most is the number of dentists that we see that don't even know they need to know occlusion. Who've never equilibrated a patient. And who have no idea that TMJ is part of dentistry—that you can't understand occlusion until you understand TMJ. Dentists don't recognize their role as physicians of the total masticatory system, because there is no other specialty of medicine that is responsible for the masticatory system.

The masticatory system that we're responsible for is the focus of a lot of oral facial pain problems that need to be diagnosed. They're quite treatable. We have methods of classifying them to know what we're dealing with, rather than just lumping everything into saying, "Oh, you have TMJ." Which is what we did for years. And then we also say, "The reason you have TMJ is because you hate your mother." You've got a psychosocial stress problem, or something that's causing you to clench in this box, and therefore you've got to get rid of whatever the problem is that's causing you all of this stress.

That isn't it at all. There is a reason for that oral-facial pain. There is a reason for the occlusion muscle. But you can't even approach it logically if you haven't understood those principles of diagnosis. We're just seeing dentists that do not have any basis at all for understanding of those things. So, everything you do in practice becomes desperate.

Do you have a favorite success quote or mantra?

Love one another. Love your neighbor. When I developed something very early in my practice, it guided me in making my decisions. I tried to figure out what is something that I can depend on to ensure that any decision that I make for a patient is the right decision?

I came up with the WIDIOM rule. *Would I do it on me?* I've taught that ever since the early 60s, when evidence should follow the WIDIOM rule. If you wouldn't do it on you, then don't do it on a patient. Would you want a dentist working on you that didn't know how to properly diagnose or treat a problem? The WIDIOM rule would say, no we wouldn't.

If I'm looking at every patient that comes in, as a store full of commodities for me to sell them, then I'm going to go in there and see, okay, how many fillings? How many crowns? It's going to be a totally different deal than if my thought process is, how can I help you get a healthy mouth, that you can keep healthy and comfortable all of your life?

If that's my goal for you, and you say, "Well, you know, I don't have a whole lot of money." You say to them, "Let's figure out the best way for you to get a healthy mouth in a way that you can do it."

I don't want to create a problem for you that's bigger than the problem that you have in your mouth. I will always sit down—it didn't matter. We had a rule to see every patient. I abhor this idea of classifying patients which are worthy of you.

Most people are teaching to get rid of the ones that aren't going to be a good patient. Every patient is entitled to know what they should do to get a healthy mouth. I can't tell them that if I don't know. I don't find any resistance in patients if I approach them as though I am consulting them in making the right decisions for them.

I've got to show them their problems before they will understand that they have a need. I can show them if a tooth is loose, I can show them when they have worn through enamel into dentin...and the dentin is going to wear 7 times faster than the enamel that they've already gone through.

I can show them pus coming out under the gum; they don't see those things. Those are signs. If I don't do a thorough examination, I'm not going to be able to tell them what they need to do to keep their mouth open.

Doctors say, "Yeah, but what if you spend all of that time and then they don't do it?"

My response would be, "Which of your patients don't deserve to know that they have a problem?" From a Christian viewpoint, I look at you and say, "My job is to love you and do the best I can to help you have the best you can have." There are a lot of patients that come in with very limited funds. Okay then, how can we work out the best thing for you? We may have to compromise, but the compromises of today, will often allow us to patch up a mouth and hold it together. We do a crown a year sometimes, that's all.

In regards to your dental career, what would you like your legacy to be, or how would you like to be remembered?

I want dentists to know, they can practice with total integrity, with fair fees, and doing it with a schedule that permits them to have balance in their family life by knowing when enough is enough. They can make all they need to live a very, very good life. Once you have enough to live a good life, every time you add on patients at the end of the day, and all of this, you're taking time away from the family.

Know when enough is enough...contentment. The enemy of contentment is comparison. If you think, "Well, there is this guy down the street making twice as much as I'm making, then I need to make that much,"—you're never going to be satisfied. Don't worry about that stuff.

What is your morning routine (first 1–2 hrs of the day)?

I get up and the first thing I do is Bible study. Probably for a good hour every day. Yup. It makes my day.

How long have you done that?

Probably a few years now. I teach a men's Bible study to about 25 men. Then I teach Sunday School, and so, you know, I have extra reason to study more. I have a bunch of commentaries that I go through. I study the Bible deeply, other than just superficially. Every day it helps me to have a joyful life.

For many years, I got up and ran the 5 miles before I went to work. I don't do that anymore. I do as much exercising as I can, but I'm 87 years old. I'm content with walking and playing golf. I also read a lot.

My wife has Alzheimer's, and she's in a nursing home, in Highland. It's only 5 minutes from where our home is. I go see her every day and spend time with her. And that's a joy; she still knows who I am. I feel very joyful in my life, even with my wife being ill and all of that.

What is your biggest fear?

I have zero fears. It's biblical: Dismiss all anxiety. Trust the Lord. Let go and let God. I have an eternal perspective. I know where I'm going when I die. And I firmly believe that.

Please explain the most challenging time in your career and how you moved past it and thrived on the other side?

I call it the curse of the entrepreneur, because I have entrepreneurial tendencies. I can visualize and so it becomes a game when I visualize something and figure out a way to make it happen, and we can often feel like we want to do it. I ended up in real estate; I built up a 15-story office building, where we put our practice in. I set up a bank and got involved with that. Got involved with a lot of stuff. Ended up with my life out of balance, because I had too many extracurricular activities.

I never did those things because I particularly wanted to be rich...it's like a challenge, you know? Every one of those things you do takes time. You end up not having the time to spend with your family like you should, and I didn't need all of those extracurricular activities.

Now I would do a better job concentrating on what I do best, and that's practicing dentistry and teaching. So, I got rid of all of those extracurricular activities, and then decided that I had a full-time career practicing, and full-time career teaching, because by then I opened the Dawson Academy.

That all took a lot of time. It was keeping that organized, plus some-how lecturing, and writing books, and all of that. I said, "Well, when is enough, enough?" I decided that "either/or" was my rule. I can either continue to practice and do all of this, or if I concentrate on just one, or the other, I could do a better job.

Well, I felt like if I put all of my concentration on teaching, that would have a multiplier effect. I practiced enough years and restored enough mouths, several thousand, and probably tens of thousands of equilibra-tions. I needed to concentrate on teaching, and I turned my practice over to my partners. I had 4 partners. I devoted 100% of my time to teaching.

When I did that, I found time—now, I could spend a whole summer in North Carolina, play some golf, and have time to think and time to write. I ended up writing another book, and designing another seminar. I could use the time to do a better job of teaching, and still have my summers free.

What is your goal-setting process?

You have to decide—you have to decide what your vision is. I developed this block scheduling, and did a lot of work on the basis that your schedule controls your life as a dentist.

I also developed what's called a practice matrix. You decide the designators of time within which you want to practice, and that means what time you want to go to work, what time you want to close up, what days you want to work. That's your practice matrix.

Then you concentrate on the time you decided within that framework, how do I get more efficient? More effective? You do that by training your staff better, having the best equipment you can have, the best procedures. It's amazing. This eliminates a lot of wasted time, which we see is so common in a dental practice.

I became tremendously productive without stress, because with block scheduling, I never scheduled more patients than I could see. It was designed to give me all of the time I needed to do the best job possible. Everything is related to planning, organizing, and thinking things through.

What is the best investment you have made either inside your career or outside of dentistry?

The best investment, by far, has been my dental practice. I never cut any corners on that. See, I realized this entrepreneurial tendency that I had, getting into all of these extracurricular things. I realized, you know, that's time and money spent that I could devote to my practice.

Any dentist who does dentistry well, does not need extracurricular sources. You need to put money aside, starting early on, for your retirement. You need a power account for building up funds when you want something. I followed a principal that said, any luxury item I want, I will pay cash for.

Looking back, what advice would you give yourself on the day of your dental school graduation?

When you graduate from dental school, I think of that as now you have an opportunity to learn to become a dentist. Unless there is some exception that we have totally missed, they're not ready to become a dentist when they get out of school. Because we don't see—we see almost nobody being trained in occlusion. If someone has not been trained in occlusion, they don't know how to even diagnose when what you're looking at is an occlusion problem.

So, a good example is, a patient goes to the local dentist. That dentist makes them a crown on their CAD machine. Then that patient comes back because now they've got these headaches, a toothache, or some kind of pain in the face.

And then, the dentist says, "Well, it isn't anything that I've done."

And the patient says, "Well, I didn't have that until you put that crown in."

The dentist says, "Well, it will take you a little while to get used to it."

That patient is going to come back several times complaining, saying they're still not feeling better. It's getting worse. And the next thing you know, we think it's an abscessed tooth. So, we'll take the tooth out. The patient didn't have an abscessed tooth; they had an occlusion problem. And with the new materials and the new CAD CAM technologies, dentists are able to screw up mouths faster, if they don't have the fundamentals. And we don't see them having the fundamentals that they need to practice in a way that is completely predictable.

So, if we want to have a happy and successful practice that you're enjoying, then we have to think of it in terms of, "How predictable is what I'm doing going to be for my patients?" You can have total predictability, everything is learnable, the processes are there. We can teach the dentist everything they need to know, through first of all, proper diagnosis, proper treating planning.

If they don't know that, they don't even know that they're the ones causing a lot of the problems. And that covers whether it's general dentistry, putting in a crown that's high, or doing orthodontics, where they get the upper teeth straight and the lower teeth straight, but when they come together, they have no relationship to the TMJ.

Predictability allows you to do your dentistry, put it in, have it perfect, and go on to the next patient. Whereas putting it in and then having to grind on it, and rework it, and reshape it, and remake it, and then having the patients come back—that wastes time while you could be seeing the other patient. So, although predictability is a buzzword, it's the first thing.

I don't understand the reluctance, of young dentists getting out of school, to do very high-quality post-graduate education. The ones that are doing that are thriving. The dentists that are coming through our Dawson Academy are just going so far ahead of the usual and customary dentists, they're not even in the same league.

They'll say, "I can't afford to do it." What they don't understand is that any time they go to a good post-graduate course, if they learn one thing, it would really help them improve what they're doing. They're going to be doing that every day, for the rest of their practice. Yet, they'll sit there and putz through trying to—let's see if—let's try this and see if it works, and then have a patient back in and grinding, and adjusting, and all, because they didn't know how to do it right in the first place. So, the first step then is to learn how to do dentistry right.

Not knowing how is very frustrating, it's stressful, and it's very unsatisfying. They don't get the reward of the fulfillment that a dentist gets who can properly diagnose and treat with successful results. This is a huge difference, as you can imagine. It's available; it's a matter of just learning how to do things that you weren't taught to do, or maybe you were taught to do them wrong.

Second thing is they have to have realistic expectations and know when enough is enough. You can make a very good living, practicing dentistry the way it should be practiced. There are a lot of practice management gurus who are leaving you with the impression that the best practice management advice is to get as many patients as you can into your practice, and sell them as much dentistry as you can.

We take a Christian viewpoint on every patient, of every patient. I love them enough to be their advocate. A big mistake most dentists make is selling commodities. In other words, they're thinking, "How many crowns can I sell this patient?", "Can I sell this patient X-rays? Can I sell this patient an exam?". That's the wrong mindset. It's not about what you CAN do, it's about what the patient's concerns are. That doesn't mean that we give the patient exactly what they say they want, because the patient doesn't know what they need.

And so, the best practices start out with a complete examination. What's the usual and customary practice do? A 15-minute exam with a sharp explorer and 2 bitewings. If they knew the difference, they would see that as malpractice. Because our job as an honest dentist is to be an advocate, and to help every patient.

See, our job is to help every patient have a healthy mouth. And how are we going to do that if we don't do a complete examination to start with, so that we know what their problems are? And what are the implications of not treating that problem in a timely way? Because every dental problem we have is progressive.

In your opinion, what separates the top 10% of dentists from the bottom 90%?

I had a seminar which was called, "How to Put Your Practice Into the Top 10%."

Absolutely number one: proper, complete exam on every new patient. No exceptions. Now, if a patient comes in for an emergency toothache, of course, you're going to take care of that. But you're also going to proceed on with setting up for figuring out why did they get into this mess in the first place?

Always do the least amount of dentistry you have to do, to get the patient's mouth healthy.

What is the best business advice you ever received?

Best business advice would be, don't spend more than you make. That's number one. Try to eliminate that as fast as you can. In other words, don't go out and try to load up on a lot of luxuries when you've got a heavy debt. Pay the debt off first.

Don't feel like you've got to keep up with the Jones' when you got to go out and borrow a ton of money to have the biggest house in the neighborhood. If you do well in dentistry, you'll be able to afford the biggest house. But don't do it until you can do it.

What leadership advice would you give a dentist who has an ineffective culture in their practice?

Number one, you learn how to do everything we teach the staff to do. In other words, you learn how to pour it up so you can show your staff. You learn how to make provisionals, so you can show them how to do it. If you need to, you can have other people come in to help you learn, and help your staff learn.

What advice would you give a dentist that is struggling with case acceptance?

Well, they're trying to sell a commodity. When a patient understands a problem, by showing them that they've worn through the enamel, showing them pus coming out from under the gum, or a loose tooth, they will often accept treatment.

With dentists who say, "My patients resist." It's only because they're trying to sell patients stuff that they don't understand.

I wouldn't ask a patient, did they want an exam. I never had anybody object to it. The number one time when patients send other people to your practice, is at the end of the first appointment. They say, "Well, I've never had such thoroughness. I'd never had a dentist sit down and explain things to me."

Dentists need to be saying:

Let me help you understand what's going on here...

Let me help you understand why we're saying this...

Look in the mirror and see that you've worn all of the enamel off, let me help you understand why that's important to you...

What marketing advice would you give a dentist that is starting out in practice ownership?

There is one thing a dentist can do; it's the most important thing they can do for building a really fine practice, and it's the one thing that people skip. Do you know what that is?

A complete examination, a perio exam, a check of occlusion, and checking the joints.

Problems are going to be progressive if we don't stop them early and diagnose the cause of the problem. But that's what dentists want to skip, and instead they put these ads in, to come in for 2 bitewings and a 15-minute exam.

What do our dental patients most desire?

Every patient wants a healthy mouth. Secondly, they want a nice-look-ing mouth. They may tell you, "I don't care what it looks like. I just want to feel more comfortable." Trust me, they care what it looks like. I've had patients say, "Look, I don't care. I just want to get out of pain." You put those new provisionals in there, they look like a million dollars, and one wife says, "He can't walk past the storefront without looking at the reflection."

Every patient wants a healthy mouth. When they call and say, "All I want is my teeth cleaned." Why do they do that? Because that's the only thing they know to ask for. They wouldn't be coming in to get their teeth cleaned if they didn't think that was the way to keep their teeth.

There are so many misconceptions about what patients want. Patients are far more responsive to understanding the reason for a good bite than most dentists are. Because patients don't have to unlearn a lot of stuff.

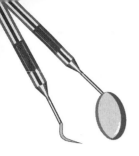

DR. STEPHANIE ZELLER

Dental Outliers Podcast,
Prosthodontist

Background

Stephanie Zeller DDS,MS practices as a prosthodontist in Seattle, WA. After graduating from dental school at the University of Missouri-Kansas City, she practiced general dentistry for several years in Kansas and New Mexico while simultaneously accumulating hundreds of hours of continuing education.

She then returned to school and acquired a Master's degree along with a specialty certificate in prosthodontics from Baylor College of Dentistry in Dallas, TX. While in her residency, she was the recipient of a research grant and an award for her research in digital dentistry. Since then, she has lectured all over the country on digital dentistry and worked with various companies to further development.

Her clinical special interests include cosmetic dentistry, implant dentistry and guided surgery, digital dentistry, and dental photography. Dr. Zeller focuses her time on lecturing, treating patients, research, publishing, collaborating, and podcasting.

Please explain your style of practice (practice size, location, procedure mix, etc.)

Seattle, Washington...prosthodontic practice. Predominantly prosthodontic procedures including full mouth reconstructions, implant dentistry, cosmetic dentistry.

Do you have a favorite success quote or mantra?

"Without change there is no innovation, creativity or incentive for improvement. Those who initiate change will have a better opportunity to manage the change that is inevitable."

—WILLIAM POLLARD

"Creativity is allowing yourself to make mistakes. Art is knowing which ones to keep."

—SCOTT ADAMS

In regards to your dental career, what would you like your legacy to be, or how would you like to be remembered?

I would like to be remembered as someone who was not afraid of change, who was willing to test limits, who fought for a predictable evolution of the craft, who sought to encourage and empower others, and who lived as authentically and as bravely as possible.

What does success mean to you?

For me, success is not one thing, but something that can exist from moment to moment. If you are living in a state of growth, doing all that you can to express your true self, including your love and creativity, then regardless of societal status or monetary gain, I would consider you, in the moment, successful.

What is your morning routine (first 1–2 hrs of the day)?

Wake up typically around 4:30am. Make coffee. Read for 30–45 minutes. Do morning pages for about 20 minutes (re: see book *Artist's Way* for morning pages). Meditation for 5–20 minutes. Shower, get ready, leave for work.

What is your biggest fear?

My biggest fear is losing my sense of self, and thus wasting the moments of my one precious life.

Please explain the most challenging time in your career and how you moved past it and thrived on the other side?

When I first started out in practice after dental school, I came up against several obstacles, including slow practice growth at multiple locations due to moving several times.

As tempting as it was to get down on myself, I took a great deal of time then to learn. I read multiple books and took online and in-person courses for dentistry, and I also read books on marketing and societal influence and learned about social media when it first came out. In return, I ended up going back to school to become a prosthodontist, which has lead to an extreme sense of gratification. It also led to a thorough understanding of social media, which I have since excelled at, and it helped me to grow my clinical practice, public profile, and lecturing career.

What is your goal-setting process?

I have a very unique perspective on goal-setting, which I have found to be not very relatable to the masses. The only goals that I usually set are short-term. I will typically verbalize these or write them down, and am usually able to achieve them.

In contrast, I rarely set long-term goals. I have found that, in concert with setting long term goals, expectations are unintentionally made in unison. There are multiple problems with expectations. First, they can potentially limit us. If we have one idea of how life should go in our minds, and we are only focused on that, our gaze may be so fixed that we miss out on other, potentially more worthwhile pursuits that might require us to relinquish our goal and pivot.

Secondly, a failure of our expectations to come to fruition may result in suffering. As Jeff Bezos said, "Expectations, not outcomes, govern the happiness of your perceived reality." Because of this, I try to avoid long-term goals and expectations, which I believe has provided me with a greater capacity to pivot often.

Dave: *This perspective is so interesting. No doubt there are times when I made myself miserable chasing poorly-engineered goals. Generally, it was because I was clear on "what" the goal was but not clear on "why" I was pursuing it (or the why was shallow). I've definitely experienced more joy since I have given more focus to morning routines and winning the day.*

What is the best investment you have made either inside your career or outside of dentistry?

DSLR. Microscope for microscope dentistry.

Looking back, what advice would you give yourself on the day of your dental school graduation?

If you decide to go in with a private practice or corporation as an associate, be very clear and thorough with the people you intend to work with. Set clear goals and expectations of both parties, and set a time to converse about progress.

Make sure that communication is accessible and open. Also, do market research in your area before accepting compensation to assure it is fair.

In your opinion, what separates the top 10% of dentists from the bottom 90%?

Mindset. A mindset for desired growth often leads to increased learning, greater knowledge to leverage, and an accelerated rate of return, including joy within one's career and monetary gain.

What keeps struggling dentists struggling?

Lack of knowledge.

What are the top 3 books every dental practice owner should read?

Mastery by Robert Greene
The Obstacle is the Way by Ryan Holiday
Thinking Fast and Slow by Daniel Kahneman

If you had to narrow it down to a couple...what traits or skills do you think are most important in running an uncommonly successful practice?

The capacity to connect with people, including good listening skills and conversational skills. Empathy. Attention to detail in regards to the business. Not micro-managing staff.

Justin: *I think Stephanie nailed this answer. The capacity to connect with people is what sets us apart.*

What is a skill or procedure you've added since graduating from dental school that has had a major positive impact on your practice?

Dental photography. Also, a thorough understanding of the complexities of diagnostics, particularly in large and complex implant surgical cases.

What is the best business advice you ever received?

If you don't know, wait.

Remain open and the answers will present themselves with time.

What leadership advice would you give a dentist who has an ineffective culture in their practice?

Bringing a mediator into the practice can be helpful. Also, making sure you have the right people for the job—if they aren't, be willing to let them go. It's best not just for you, but for the staff and even for the person you are letting go.

Dave: Having the right people for the job is a great topic. As a leader, oftentimes I wanted someone's success more than they did. I saw potential in them that they didn't. I was hard on myself because I couldn't get them to the next level.

However, I've come to the realization that there are things that are nearly impossible to teach: work ethic, values, attention to detail, etc. Some of your biggest wins in practice will come at the point of hire. Unfortunately, it sometimes takes awhile to determine if it's a win or not.

What advice would you give a dentist that is struggling with case acceptance?

Find someone that has a high acceptance rate and present a mock case to them. Be open to their feedback.

Justin: This is a great actionable tip!

What marketing advice would you give a dentist that is starting out in practice ownership?

Your best referrals come from other patients. Focus on the experience for the patients at the beginning, even if it takes extra time. It's worth it.

What do our dental patients most desire?

A good experience, and someone that cares about them and listens to them.

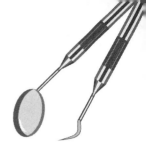

DR. ANDREW TURCHIN

Cosmetic Confidence Coaching

Background

I grew up in the Tri-State Area in a middle class family as great and as imperfect as the next. My father was a very hard-working CPA/CFO who urged me not to work for anyone else, having made others so much money over the years.

I went to Rutgers Undergrad and UMDNJ(now Rutgers) Dental School, followed by an AEGD at Columbia. I always knew in dental school that I wanted to do quality dentistry; I just didn't quite know what that meant at the time. I later found that to mean a good understanding of occlusion, facial esthetics, and natural beauty.

After AEGD, I was lucky enough to land an associate position at a well-known prosthodontics clinic on Fifth Avenue. After 2.5 years, I stupidly hung a shingle and did some moonlighting for Larry Rosenthal on the side. Eventually, I bought a small practice and grew my NYC practice into a great practice. And when I had my dream practice, I said goodbye to NYC to move to Aspen, CO and follow my dreams of being a professional ski bum.

In the 5 years since we moved to Aspen, we have built a practice that rivals my NYC practice, and we treat patients from all over the country and world with a focus on cosmetics, occlusion, and how it all plays a role in facial esthetics. I've developed the Anti-Aging Smile™ and teach other dentists how to diagnose, present, and predictably perform these cosmetic dental procedures.

Dave: *Andrew's temps look better than most doctor's permanent veneers. I admire his dedication to clinical excellence. But the thing that I most respect him for is his courage to walk away from an outstanding cosmetic practice in New York City and pursue the lifestyle he dreamed of. There were many naysayers that said he couldn't do what he has done in Aspen. I appreciate people who prove the consensus wrong and go after what they want.*

Please explain your style of practice (practice size, location, procedure mix, etc.)

I have a 4-op office in Aspen, CO that we are currently moving to a new location with 5 ops, photo studio, porcelain lab, and 2 consult rooms.

Do you have a favorite success quote or mantra?

If you think you can, you're probably right. If you think you cannot, you are definitely right.

In regards to your dental career, what would you like your legacy to be, or how would you like to be remembered?

I would like to be remembered by my patients for improving smiles and slowing down and reversing the aging process. I would also like to be remembered by dentists for giving them the confidence to do the same for patients by making the clinical diagnosis and treatment simpler and more predictable.

What does success mean to you?

Success to me is being happy and enjoying life. For me, that's time with my wife Gina, daughter Ava, and skiing.

What is your morning routine (first 1–2 hrs of the day)?

My morning routine is boring. I am not a morning person. I love playing with Ava for a bit before getting to the office for our morning huddle.

What is your biggest fear?

My biggest fear is that the big cases stop coming. I've built up the capacity and capabilities to handle those big cases, in addition to my enjoying them; so it would not be fun if they slowed down. And since I don't do any external marketing, I don't feel like I have that dial to control my NP volume. Luckily, I love talking about what I do, am relatively social, and built up a reputation. So, that seems to be working.

Justin: This answer really resonated with me. I really appreciated the vulnerability. I mean it's easy for us all to say "my fear is that I won't be able to help enough people", which may be true for a few people, ie. Mother Theresa. But let's be honest, if you are a practice owner, most of us at least at times will deep down have that feeling of "what if?". What if this crumbles? What if the patients stop coming in? What if this gravy train derails? Not that you or I wouldn't pick ourselves up, make the necessary pivots, and do what we need to do; but who wants to be forced to make those decisions if we don't have to? If I am going to make a life change or reinvent myself, I'd much prefer to make the choice on my terms in my time, not because the dentistry stopped coming in. Great answer, IMO.

Please explain the most challenging time in your career and how you moved past it and thrived on the other side?

My most challenging time in my career was losing most of my team all at one time, and I mean everyone except my hygienist. I was down from 3 dental assistants to 0 and no one at the front. I was away in Italy and didn't want to tell my wife to ruin her time as well, but I was a mess inside. I was scared and it made me doubt myself as a leader. I emailed my last front desk person and told her my fears, my doubts, and my desperation. She responded with all the support I could have ever asked for. She said she'd be back part time (she left to start her own business); she reminded me of how much I had accomplished, and how much I taught her. She gave me the confidence when I was doubting myself. We managed to dig up some temps to come to my small town; my long-time dental assistant from NYC moved to Aspen for 3 months to get us back on our feet and help train someone new.

It's hard to imagine, but this wasn't the first or the last time this has happened. I live in a transient resort town and quality team members or people with dental experience are hard to find. After years of stability on my team in NYC, I am getting used to the new normal of always looking for and training new team members. I'd rather not, but it's the price to pay for living in my dream location.

Dave: *Wow. Andrew's response puts a pit in my stomach. Also practicing in a small resort town, I've taken out more Craigslist ads than I want to admit. Good team members that will stick around are so difficult to find. It's a perpetual leadership test in many of these mountain ski communities.*

What is your goal-setting process?

I'm a thinker, so I can't help but think about and envision my goals relatively regularly. I don't mean that I have a set schedule or anything, but I do something I call dreamscaping 1–2 times per year when I am on a plane without a baby. Something about being locked into that seat for a bunch of hours has always made the time my most productive. I am always reading or writing or both on a plane.

Dreamscaping is a simple exercise of writing your goals down and then figuring out how to make them happen. As many have heard me speak, one of my guiding principles is to "Begin with the End in Mind" when it comes to clinically, practice management, and in my life. So this is a way to Begin with the End, and then back it into the schedule. Let's say you feel like you're relatively busy in the office producing $800K and can't imagine how you'll ever grow bigger. Or you're doing a startup and want to make some goals but don't know where to start, or you're not sure if you believe you can do X.

Let's take that busy $800K practice and say you want to grow it to $1.2MM next year. Yes, I said $1.2MM. Why not? Probably because someone told you to think in term of 5% growth. Well, that's not growth, that's inflation. Goals should be 20–50% growth unless you're where you want to be.

So, you write down $1.2MM and then draw up a schedule for your ideal day—nothing crazy or impossible. Hygiene, op1, op2, should I start using my 3rd op? Do I need another assistant? Can I run that third chair for assistant-driven production such as Invisalign, nightguards, whitening, etc.? The brainstorming is beginning. Actually block off each new patient appointment so that you'll have enough capacity for your current NP flow (or the one you might need to get to your goal), and the same with the rest of your procedure mix. Don't forget inserts, and post ops, and such. Then add up the production for each column/chair and multiply by number of days.

The number might surprise you. It's often as high or higher than your goal. So what does this fictitious exercise prove to you? First and foremost, that you can do that number and thus give you the confidence you need. Secondly, it gives you a clear picture of how to produce that 50% more. And lastly, it gives you some pretty good idea of what you'll need to do to get you there—ie. equip extra op, another assistant, increase my clinical efficiency, increase NP's, etc.

Dreamscaping might sound silly, but it has in it many great attributes. It gives you vision, it builds confidence, and it gives you much of the direction or sub-goals that need to happen. And it's served me very well over the years.

What is the best investment you have made either inside your career or outside of dentistry?

The best investment I have made in my career would have to be my associateships in the beginning of my career. Having worked for Jonathon Levine, having as my mentor Jeffrey McClendon (another dentist in his office), spending time in their lab, and then associating with Larry Rosenthal, I gained knowledge and experience that was not teachable in a course. It's why I believe so strongly in the apprentice or mentor model that I am bringing back to dentistry.

Looking back, what advice would you give yourself on the day of your dental school graduation?

Find as many mentors as you can in life and learn with abandon.

In your opinion, what separates the top 10% of dentists from the bottom 90%?

Focus and drive. They might focus on different things, but they are focused.

Justin: I would add to this that focusing on the "right" things is a separation indicator. We all have a limited amount of focus. Some may have more, some may have less, but it's all finite. Being able to narrow the focus on the things that really move the needle in a dental practice, I believe, is imperative for uncommon success.

What keeps struggling dentists struggling?

A lack of confidence that they can do it—whatever "it" is. Whether it's drop insurance, or do a complex case, or ski a few days per week.

What are the top 3 books every dental practice owner should read?

The 7 Habits of Highly Effective People by Stephen Covey
The Big Leap by Gay Hendricks
The Checklist Manifesto by Atul Gawande

If you had to narrow it down to a couple...what traits or skills do you think are most important in running an uncommonly successful practice?

That's a tough one, because there are so many different people who succeed. The gift of gab gets some people there. Leadership stands out, though, as most important. We need to lead our patients and our team.

Dave: Leadership thought leader, John Maxwell has his "Law of the Lid". It states that leadership ability determines a person's level of effectiveness. It's a strong statement. But in my opinion, too many dentists ignore leadership as their responsibility. In denying that they need to lead and what the multiplying effects of good leadership are, they struggle more than need be.

What is a skill or procedure you've added since graduating from dental school that has had a major positive impact on your practice?

First, ideal occlusion and esthetics. More recently, sleep apnea.

What is the best business advice you ever received?

Begin With The End in Mind.

What leadership advice would you give a dentist who has an ineffective culture in their practice?

Time to have some honest conversations with yourself and your team. Maybe you need help leading—I prefer to have a co-leader on the team.

What advice would you give a dentist that is struggling with case acceptance?

Don't tell patients what they "need". People don't like being told what to do.

What marketing advice would you give a dentist that is starting out in practice ownership?

Internal marketing has been the most effective for me. So don't be shy about your differentiating factors.

What do our dental patients most desire?

Longevity and lack of emergencies.

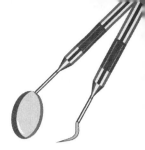

DR. JASON OLITSKY

Smile Stylist, Clinical Mastery

Justin: *I've known Jason and his wife Colleen for many years, dating back to our time working with Dr. Blatchford. I've attended his courses at Clinical Mastery, and can say when it comes to cosmetic dentistry and photography, this guy has got it going on. If I was in the market for a new smile, the Smile Stylist is who I would go to. He also has the coolest practice website that I've seen. Check it out: www.TheSmileStylist.com*

Background

Jason Olitsky, DMD AAACD, a 2001 graduate of Temple University School of Dentistry, is past president of the Florida Academy of Cosmetic Dentistry and an accredited member of the American Academy of Cosmetic Dentistry.

He is the Program Director for The Clinical Mastery Series. He teaches portrait and clinical photography and over-the-shoulder anterior aesthetics courses with The Clinical Mastery Series. He is on the Editorial Review Board of Inside Dentistry. He is also a KOL with Digital Smile Design. He is a clinical consultant with Dental Advisor. He publishes on various topics of cosmetic dentistry, has appeared in numerous national beauty and health magazines, and serves as product consultant for dental product companies.

He maintains a private practice in Ponte Vedra Beach, Florida with his wife Colleen Olitsky.

From Jason: I am an avid soccer player. I currently play on two adult soccer teams throughout the year. Growing up, I played for the state of Florida in Olympic development. I also enjoy surfing. I have traveled to Central America many times to surf. I actually chose my current practice location close to the beach, partly so I could surf more often.

Please explain your style of practice (practice size, location, procedure mix, etc.)

We opened our practice in 2006 as a start-up. I have a 3-chair dental practice. Two restorative chairs and one for hygiene. We opened our practice in 2006 as a cosmetic practice with a focus on smile design. Our niche is a hip youthful atmosphere and the bulk of our clientele is 20s, 30s, 40s, and 50s; however we perform a good amount of cosmetic dentistry for patients outside that range. Focusing on a younger vibe in the office keeps our style unique and current. I have a full photo studio in the practice to take pictures of new patients, consultations, procedures, and after pictures. Current marketing efforts in dentistry are very visual with social media and internet and it helps to have excellent photography and video capabilities in the practice.

Do you have a favorite success quote or mantra?

"If you are not willing to risk the usual,
you will have to settle for the ordinary."

—JIM ROHN

It is easy to be ordinary in dentistry. You can be ordinary and have a great income, take care of your family, and have a successful practice. To change things, we have to have a strong vision for our future, then have to risk the ordinary and work towards realizing our ideal vision.

In regards to your dental career, what would you like your legacy to be, or how would you like to be remembered?

He pushed us harder to realistically achieve more natural results and improved our mindset for what is possible for digital documentation. I really cared about improving the lives of dentists through helping increase their passion for dentistry and living their lives to the fullest. We have an amazing profession, helping dentists to their fullest potential and to realize their professional and personal goals.

What does success mean to you?

"Success is doing what you want to do,
when you want, where you want,
with whom you want, as much as you want."

−TONY ROBBINS

What is your morning routine (first 1–2 hrs of the day)?

Gym days, up at 5:00am. Come home at 6:00am. Answer emails and catch up on work. Kids up between 6:30–7:00am. Help get kids ready for school. Walk with them to bus stop or drive them to school. 8:15am work. First patient at 9:00am.

What is your biggest fear?

Drowning.

Please explain the most challenging time in your career and how you moved past it and thrived on the other side?

We received an advertising violation from the Florida Board of Dentistry about 4 months into our new practice. We were turned in by a fellow dentist in our area for laudatory comments which were subjective in nature and also used by a good amount of other dentists in our city. The fine was hefty, but it was also disheartening that a fellow local dentist had an extreme distaste for us and the change that we brought to our area. Why were we singled out among all the other dentists who advertised in our city? Risking a second violation would mean disciplinary action against our license. We had to completely change our advertising.

The adversity led to a complete rebrand, the birth of Smile Stylist, and our influence to change an industry. Today we are licensing Smile Stylist to qualified dentists who want to increase their leads and case acceptance for cosmetic dentistry treatments.

Dave: *Reminds me of a Napoleon Hill quote that I lean on during challenging times: "Every adversity, every failure, every heartache carries with it the seed of an equal or greater benefit."*

What is your goal-setting process?

I write down my goals and visualize my goals. I have a very strong vision about what I want to accomplish in my professional career, and I work hard to realize my potential. I firmly believe that it is not the talent or the artistry or skill of the dentist, but the relentless drive to accomplish, that will provide the results we are looking to achieve.

Justin: *I'm glad Jason touched on the visualization aspect. We always hear to write our goals down, but not nearly as often do we hear to visualize ourselves with the end result. What's going to be different once the goals written down are accomplished? How will that sense of pride make you feel? How will your life be improved? If the end goal is grand enough, the work required to get there becomes irrelevant.*

What is the best investment you have made either inside your career or outside of dentistry?

The best investments I have made are in continuing education, focused on realization of my vision. Investment with a practice management coach and techniques to perform the dentistry and personal growth have been important financial and time investments, but also investing time in my personal relationships with my wife and children at home. I invest the time into letting my dental team know I appreciate them and what they do for me and our patients. Balance is very important to me and I can tell when my life is not in balance. I invest in balance.

Looking back, what advice would you give yourself on the day of your dental school graduation?

Start out by focusing on improving the motor skills and treatment-planning knowledge necessary to be a great dentist. Do a lot of dentistry. Then determine a path for your career, find your passion, and make conscious decisions that align yourself with the path. Determine what you want your practice to be like in ten years, then create it right away. Invest in your CE.

In your opinion, what separates the top 10% of dentists from the bottom 90%?

Laser-like focus on what you want your practice to be like. The top 10% of dentists are just like the other 90%, but they have momentum for success. If you really want something, you will find the way; if you don't, then you will find the excuse.

What keeps struggling dentists struggling?

You get what you tolerate.

What are the top 3 books every dental practice owner should read?

1   A book that is written about real successful practices. Modeling is the quickest pathway to success.

2   *The Millionaire Next Door* by Thomas Stanley

3   *The Answer* by John Assaraf

4   *Integrity Selling for the 21st Century* by Ron Willingham

If you had to narrow it down to a couple...what traits or skills do you think are most important in running an uncommonly successful practice?

Innovation, Marketing, Determination.

What is a skill or procedure you've added since graduating from dental school that has had a major positive impact on your practice?

Occlusion. Preparation and cementation of all ceramic materials. Talking to patients to connect and asking the right questions. Photography. Photography provides us an opportunity to make emotional connections with our customers.

What is the best business advice you ever received?

Oren Harari in *Break From The Pack* wrote, I paraphrase, that in order to consistently win a race, you need to run your own race. Stop running the same race as everyone else. Create your own category and and dominate!

What leadership advice would you give a dentist who has an ineffective culture in their practice?

Leader attitude is reflected in the team. Start with yourself. Fix your attitude, then expect it from your team.

What advice would you give a dentist that is struggling with case acceptance?

In order to increase case acceptance, we need to increase our enthusiasm for the treatments. Enthusiasm comes from confidence.

Confidence comes from being successful at providing the treatments, making patients happy, and having experience and knowledge in the treatments performed for the patients.

For cosmetic dentistry, it is important to have a portfolio of work to show patients. When a dentist is new to cosmetic dentistry, it is OK to discount services to help increase case acceptance. It is part of education, gaining experience and confidence, and building a portfolio. Make sure to take excellent pictures to document for a portfolio. Get a good model release for your patients and have them sign releases in exchange for discounted services. Get your product out there! The other side of case acceptance is your communication with the patient.

What marketing advice would you give a dentist that is starting out in practice ownership?

We started marketing our startup practice at 10% of our projected production. Today, social media has created a marketing outlet that reduces our total costs of marketing and allows us to share information in real time. Understand social media marketing and get good at taking pictures and videos to share.

What do our dental patients most desire?

That we understand and respect their values.

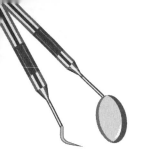

DR. LANE OCHI

Beverly Hills Cosmetic Dentist

Background

Dr. Ochi graduated with honors from the University of Southern California in 1981, where he received the Robert W. McNulty Memorial Award for the highest scholastic achievement. He is a Fellow in the American College of Dentists and the International College of Dentists.

He is currently an Associate Clinical Professor in the Department of Restorative Dentistry, and was the Co-director of Occlusion at U.S.C. School of Dentistry. He is also an Assistant Director in the Advanced Restorative Institute Dental Education Center, on the faculty of the Esthetic Professionals Education Center, and serves as a specialist consultant to the Graduate Prosthodontic Program at the Veterans Affairs Hospital in West Los Angeles.

He has lectured to national and international audiences on the subject of aesthetic restorative dentistry and occlusion. He has received multiple Commendations from the County of Los Angeles for his efforts to promote the health and wellbeing of underserved populations in his community.

Dr. Ochi maintains a full-time private practice in Beverly Hills with an emphasis on physiologic and aesthetic reconstructive dentistry. His patients include Academy Award winners, and some of the most recognized names in the entertainment business.

His passion for competitive cycling is shared as the longest running sponsor of Velo Club La Grange, one of California's largest and oldest cycling clubs with over 400 members nationwide. Past members include a Tour de France stage winner, a racer in the 2012 Tour de France, an Olympic gold medalist, and numerous U.S. National, Mexican, and California state champions. His ongoing support for the juniors' and women's teams has allowed many members to pursue their sport and develop their skills as bike racers.

And when not on a bike, he can be found practicing the Zen of fly fishing. His travels have taken him to some of the most beautiful regions of our country, where he has achieved "grand slam" status on many waters.

Please explain your style of practice (practice size, location, procedure mix, etc.)

My practice is limited to restorative dentistry. I am located at "ground zero" for elective care, Beverly Hills, California. It is a full fee-for-service practice, with all specialty procedures referred out. This works both ways; as a referral-based model, what could be better than having a patient come to you from another specialist who already knows what they need to have done. We are also extremely blessed to have an incredibly loyal patient base in a very mobile demographic. I am now a 3-generation provider.

Do you have a favorite success quote or mantra?

Louis Pasteur: "Chance favors the prepared mind". Sudden flashes of insight rarely happen; they are the products of preparation. Solid foundations are mandatory for a successful and fulfilling career.

In regards to your dental career, what would you like your legacy to be, or how would you like to be remembered?

In my community, there are two types of doctors. Those whose identity is defined by whom they treat, and those who want to be known for what they have accomplished in their profession. I hope my legacy reflects the latter.

I take great pride in being awarded Fellowship in the American College of Dentists, long known as "the conscience of dentistry". Fellowship is bestowed for exceptional contributions to dentistry and society. I am also a Fellow in the International College of Dentists, whose motto is "recognizing service and the opportunity to serve". Fellowship is awarded for dedication to the continued progress of dentistry for the benefit of humankind.

Dave: *I can only imagine how easy it is to get wrapped up in the status game of the Beverly Hills and Hollywood elites. Dr. Ochi's intentions speak volumes for who he is as a person.*

What does success mean to you?

Success is being able to identify what your own definition of it is, and to have the maturity to understand that definition is never static as life progresses. Success is not what we do, but becoming what we want.

What is your morning routine (first 1–2 hrs of the day)?

It took me most of my adult life to understand why one of the greatest influencers, my father, woke up so early every day. The time before your day begins is quiet and uninterrupted. Time to reflect on what the new day brings and to make plans. I take this time to review the charts for the day, answer emails and correspondence, and do lab work.

Studies have clearly shown that interruptions and multitasking are major sources of clinical inefficiency and stress. Minimizing these distractions will predictably make our lives less stressful.

What is your biggest fear?

Life is about learning and reevaluation. When I got divorced, my practice was thriving, and I was living the good life. I was at the top of my game and did not realize that I had started to become entitled. I assumed that I deserved my success because of all my hard work and sacrifice; after all, it was costing me my marriage. A massive lifestyle change occurred and I learned to balance everything better, and I'm grateful for the lesson. My biggest fear is ever feeling entitled again.

Please explain the most challenging time in your career and how you moved past it and thrived on the other side?

Mine was expecting too much from myself, and feeling the immense pressure associated with it. I built a large office and was not only burning the candle at both ends, but was trying to hold myself to unsustainable expectations, and developed a need for escape in my limited down time. Having an addictive personality can be a good thing, but it can also be very dangerous. Fortunately, I recognized my actions were self-destructive and sought help before I hit bottom. Thanks to Dr. Smith and Bill Wilson, my focus is clear and my life and dentistry are better for this defining moment.

What is your goal-setting process?

I need to ask myself several questions:

- Is this goal part of my values and core beliefs?
- Can I actually achieve this goal?
- What priorities will I need to adjust to reach this goal, and more importantly, is this goal in conflict with my current goals?
- Does this goal support the person I choose to become?

Dave: *What a powerful process to determine IF a goal is worth achieving.*

What is the best investment you have made either inside your career or outside of dentistry?

Teaching. To truly be a teacher, one must always be a student. If you possess the knowledge to answer a question, as well as know when to ask a question, chances are you are current with all the rapid changes that are occurring in our profession. There is no arrival point of knowledge. There is always a deeper refinement. There is always a new innovation on knowledge that we know.

Looking back, what advice would you give yourself on the day of your dental school graduation?

I would have listened more carefully to the words of another mentor, Jack Kennedy. I will just quote him directly.

Be a lifelong student. Study not only dentistry, but read across the curriculum. Those who study and know only dentistry, after a while, become narrowly focused and stale. The best solve many of their practice and life problems through reading literature, psychology, philosophy, history and art, as well as science.

Attempt excellence on a daily basis. The key word is attempt. No one is excellent every day, including Michael Jordan; but the more you attempt excellence, the more it finds you. Excellence in dentistry has much less to do with natural talent than it has to do with the mindset that "I`m going to give it my best each day." Most who persevere can learn to play the game of dentistry at a high level, no matter their technical skills during their formal schooling.

Be willing to accept rejection. Most who practice dentistry successfully recognize that a "no" from a patient today often is a "yes" tomorrow. Plant seeds for high-quality dentistry and you will find yourself harvesting many of these seeds at a later date. Those who fear rejection routinely offer less than their best, which cheats patients out of rightfully making their own economic decisions.

Be patient. The lifetime-success race most often goes to the turtles, rarely to the rabbits. Mark Twain said, "It took me 20 years to become an overnight success." Overspending in the personal, as well as the professional, arena seems to be endemic to doctors. Financial stress often has a negative influence on professional and personal decisions. Be innovative and creative in your practice, and be conservative with your money and how you spend and invest it.

On a daily basis, try not to take yourself too seriously. Life isn't fair; it's just life. Do not beat yourself up when you don't meet your own expectations or the expectations of others, for, at times, none of us do. The most successful people in life are the ones who routinely take a chance on being something special. The real losers are the ones who never get into the game.

Justin: There is a lot of good stuff in the preceding paragraphs. If you didn't catch it, I encourage you to read it again.

In your opinion, what separates the top 10% of dentists from the bottom 90%?

The ability to communicate, and by that, I mean listen, really listen, to patients. In the 1980s, Avrom King postulated that fine dentistry was behaviorally self-limited. King meant that regardless of the dentist's technical expertise, unless they had the requisite behavioral skills to communicate—including the ability to profoundly listen to their patients—their technical skills would go largely unused.

Successful dentists do not present cases. Case presentations should be replaced with a cooperative problem identification session in which the dentist and patient attempt to discover what is happening in the patient's mouth and what can be predicted for the years ahead. Most people will ultimately choose our best and finest care.

What keeps struggling dentists struggling?

Most of our work is done alone. Getting better is not easy and there are no shortcuts. Without mentors and support, it's easy to be affected by this. If one is struggling with any aspect of our career, then look for help. Recognize we are not alone, and take that important first step because no one else will do it for you.

What are the top 3 books every dental practice owner should read?

In no particular order:

- Bob Barkley's Successful Preventive Dental Practices.
- Daniel Kahneman's Thinking Fast and Slow.
- Steven Johnson's Where Good Ideas Come From.

If you had to narrow it down to a couple...what traits or skills do you think are most important in running an uncommonly successful practice?

The most important trait for success we can possess is patience. Our world has become one of instant gratification, a world where everything is "now and fast." We seem to have lost touch with the fact that faster doesn't always equate to achieving important goals or being effective.

Just because you keep pushing on with the daily grind, it doesn't mean you are moving forward to the results you really want in your life and work. Sometimes the most powerful, effective, and beneficial thing you can do to move forward is to take a step back. Use this to reassess, review, and get a clearer perspective. This usually results in making better decisions and allows you to make sure you are on the right track to achieve your most important goals.

What is a skill or procedure you've added since graduating from dental school that has had a major positive impact on your practice?

Developing a well-rounded understanding of occlusion has had the greatest impact on how I practice. From diagnosis to treatment planning and execution, occlusion is the foundation of single tooth dentistry to full mouth reconstruction. We need to learn all we can about occlusion because we cannot diagnose what we can't see, and we can't see what we don't know.

What is the best business advice you ever received?

I was told early on by several influencers and mentors that a successful practice takes time. The first phase is "survival", followed by "growth", and then "income", and to pace your lifestyle to match. I heard each phase could last from 5–10 years, and as it turned out, I hit each phase dead center in the bell curve. Not over reaching too soon and knowing when to invest more in myself and the office paid huge dividends later.

What leadership advice would you give a dentist who has an ineffective culture in their practice?

Change is hard for all of us. Your organizational structure is what maintains the hierarchy, facilitates communication, and keeps everything running smoothly. In order to address an ineffective culture, you first need to learn to identify the cause. Many times it's us, because we have no formal training in this. I realized early on that this was not my strength and sought outside help. I learned that success tends to breed success. Everyone in the office must have the same goals, organizational pride, ambition towards being better, teamwork and communication, and creating great patient relations.

What advice would you give a dentist that is struggling with case acceptance?

I spoke to the need of really listening to what our patients are saying. For the most part, we all tend to speak too much and not listen enough. Patient care involves hearing their concerns, understanding their goals, and working with them to create choice. This is another area where we don't receive enough training as dentists and we can learn from others.

I see two main types of dental practice models; the first get as many new patients in as possible and do as much work as possible and repeat. The other is to establish patients for life, where you develop respect and trust; these patients will always need work and will typically do what you recommend.

What marketing advice would you give a dentist that is starting out in practice ownership?

Always strive to create that "wow" experience. Make sure people understand you are accepting new patients. Internal marketing is the most powerful way to build your practice. While social media will be seen by more people, our goal is to attract the friends and families of good patients, as "like attracts like".

What do our dental patients most desire?

Honesty and integrity. What people want from us goes to the core of the doctor-patient relationship. We need to listen, to care and be compassionate, and to be transparent and open with patients.

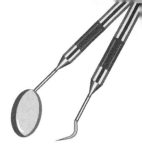

DR. STEVE VAN DE GRAAFF

Crestview Family Dental

Justin: *I've had the privilege of getting to know this next Titan over the past year or so, and I was really glad we got to include him in this book. Although I know Steve doesn't have the most "glamorous" practice, he has turned it around and made it a very strong practice that fits his personal vision.*

I don't want to steal too much of his thunder, but Steve was able to pay off $400K worth of school debt during his first year in practice, and still found time to be a solid husband and dad to their 6 kids. I find that pretty amazing, and I think he has a lot to offer here.

Background

I grew up in the Western US in a large, crazy, but happy family. I knew I wanted the same and so dentistry seemed like a profession that could get me there. I managed to get accepted into school and stayed awake enough to graduate. My wife and I enjoy our family with 6 kids. I love coaching sports, Cub Scouts, and doing anything outdoors.

I purchased a practice out of school, described briefly below, that many would consider "unique." I acquired it relatively inexpensively, have been able to serve a steady stream of new patients each month, and am fortunate to enjoy a small overhead with a strong monthly cash flow. I am not a DSO founder or a magazine-level clinician by any means. I would consider myself a very average businessman and average clinician without special gifts or uncommon talents. If anything, my story is an encouraging example of how a normal dentist with determination can do very well with the right business information and courage to follow the blueprint that others have laid out.

Please explain your style of practice (practice size, location, procedure mix, etc.)

I purchased a small practice and an old building right out of school a little over a year ago (2016). Five chairs squeezed into a very old 1300-square-foot building, located in a poor area a couple miles from other dentists. We are Medicaid, PPO, and lots of emergencies. Extractions, fillings, and pedo make up most of our production. While a majority of our patients do not accept the presented treatment of endo, crowns, or implants, we treat them great anyway and provide the treatment available to them. Our practice has a unique niche in the area for this reason, and lots of patients come to us.

Many dentists think a very successful practice must be a FFS office, or modeled around cosmetics or specialty procedures. I've discovered that while certainly not as glamorous, a lower fee and bread-and-butter practice model can be very successful as well. I've also found that it doesn't necessarily have to take many years to become profitable, build a busy practice, and pay off student loans. Ownership, coupled with clinical and business drive, have accomplished all those things for me within a year of graduation.

Do you have a favorite success quote or mantra?

Perfect is the enemy of good.

Don't piddle.

Dave: I appreciate the perfectionist nature of dentists as a whole. But as Steve points out, perfection often impedes progress.

In regards to your dental career, what would you like your legacy to be, or how would you like to be remembered?

I would hope my patients would remember me as somebody who was kind and genuinely cared about them. Simple really, doesn't even require great talent or clinical ability.

What does success mean to you?

I see clinical masters posting their impressive work online and I admire dedication to their craft.We often think of these people as the successful dentists. While I enjoy dentistry and do my best for my patients, dentistry is a means to an end for me. Success for me means having the financial freedom and freedom of time to do what I find most meaningful, which right now is being a Dad to my kids.

Dave: I honor Steve for just coming out and stating "dentistry is a means to an end" for him. I think many dentists feel guilty because they aren't super passionate about clinical dentistry. It doesn't have to stand in the way of clinical excellence or a dream practice.

What is your morning routine (first 1–2 hrs of the day)?

I confess I'm a night guy. I have a wave of energy from 9pm until midnight and usually find inspiration and efficiency during this time. In the mornings I get up at 6:30, eat oatmeal, and head off to work.

What is your biggest fear?

Letting work negatively affect my focus and success in being a father to my kids.

Please explain the most challenging time in your career and how you moved past it and thrived on the other side?

The first couple months after I bought my practice out of school, I realized there was so much I didn't understand before I jumped into the deep end of the pool that is ownership.

What to do when staff leaves. What to do when things in the office break. What to do with disappointed patients or an empty schedule. I realized I significantly overestimated my clinical ability and underestimated the difficulty of making a low-fee practice profitable.

All these challenges attached together and had me thinking that I had made a mistake in buying my practice. I had signed the loan, and there was no way out. Those couple months, to be honest, were dark times for me, emotionally and mentally. I just tried to survive, and a couple months later, things started working out.

I just kept attacking each problem every single day, and a few months later, things started going well. A year later, things are rocking and we're already doing better than I ever thought possible going in. It has been a powerful lesson in the power of belief and perseverance.

What is your goal-setting process?

Form a clear vision and image of what you want within the next several years. Map out the fastest way to get there and act quickly to put those things in motion. These actions should cause you to be uncomfortable. I recently hired a coach to help me get there faster and hold me accountable and this has been helpful.

What is the best investment you have made either inside your career or outside of dentistry?

As they say, invest in yourself. My most valuable investment was spending time learning about the business path of young dentists who became successful very early in their career.

Networking with them, asking them questions, and trying to mimic what they have done. It's nice to be in a career where we don't need to be creators or come up with profound original ideas. Just find successful dentists and copy them.

Justin: *This was one of my favorites of Steve's answers. I agree the fastest way to accomplish something is to find someone who has already accomplished what it is you want to accomplish and do what they have done.*

Looking back, what advice would you give yourself on the day of your dental school graduation?

Be careful in comparing yourself to others. Comparison is good if it inspires you to improve or change your situation for the better. Otherwise it can be a source of constant discouragement that robs you of happiness.

In your opinion, what separates the top 10% of dentists from the bottom 90%?

The most successful dentists I know all share this unrelenting drive for more. It's as if they don't consider what could go wrong. They don't wait for the right time or for when they have more experience. They just go for it, often not having all the answers or all of the plan worked out. Then, as soon as they reach their goal, they are immediately moving on to the next level, the next idea.

It's interesting; they often have very visible flaws or weaknesses like the rest of us, but they act as if they didn't. They don't procrastinate future moves or think much about past mistakes; they're just always moving forward. It's a special kind of drive. Even if this drive doesn't come naturally to you, I think we can make the same moves and be similarly successful, if we are mindful and intentional.

What keeps struggling dentists struggling?

I think fear of change. They are worried to try to do things differently. I read that 90% of our thoughts each day are reprocessed thoughts we ran through our minds the day before. It is a cycle that keeps us in a rut and throws up barriers to growth. If you're struggling with the same problems, be assertive to try something new or seek outside advice on how to change.

What are the top 3 books every dental practice owner should read?

How to Win Friends and Influence People by Dale Carnegie. Memorize the chapter headings and practice one a day.
E-Myth by Michael Gerber
Breakaway manual

If you had to narrow it down to a couple...what traits or skills do you think are most important in running an uncommonly successful practice?

Communication—Covey said this is the most important skill in life. I have found I'd rather do just about anything rather than address issues with staff and train them to change and improve. Whenever not saying something is the easy thing to do, that's when it is most important to communicate about it.

Delegation—There is no greater waste of time than doing something effectively that you don't have to do in the first place. Having assistants do everything possible, within their realm of legal activity, frees you up for more important and profitable tasks. It will also make them feel more valued and they will enjoy work more as well. It's a win-win.

Discontent—Never settle for a certain level of success. Constantly strive to reach the next level.

Justin: I found the above answer of "discontent" an interesting one. For most of my professional life, I fought against this. What I mean by that is I would regularly argue (with myself) and tell myself to just be content with where I was at. To relax, if you will.

It seemed whenever I got to a certain spot I was working to achieve, the next thing popped up out of nowhere, and I was off to the races again.

Now don't get me wrong, I do believe there has to be balance; however, I also had to come to grips with how I was wired and not give myself more grief because of who I was.

I had to come to a place where I was "content" with not being content, if that makes sense. Since I came to that realization, it has given me a lot of peace in my own life.

What is a skill or procedure you've added since graduating from dental school that has had a major positive impact on your practice?

In my fourth year of dental school, I externed at OMFS residencies and secured the opportunity to do a couple dozen thirds cases at my school as a student. I do wisdom teeth everyday now, and they are the most enjoyable and profitable procedure in my practice. No lab fee or return appointments; just a couple bucks of anesthetic and a suture. They are a practice builder for sure—lots of new patients come to me just for their wisdom teeth.

What is the best business advice you ever received?

If somebody else has done it, why can't you? Accepting this can be a large mental hurdle, but it becomes empowering once you truly believe it.

Dave: I love Steve's answer here. There are so many mental obstacles that can be cleared with the simple question: "Why not me?"

What leadership advice would you give a dentist who has an ineffective culture in their practice?

This ineffective culture likely started because staff members were not performing as they should, but the dentist was too fearful to address the situation. Learn techniques to effectively communicate with and correct a staff member. Learn how to do this even if it is awkward. Learn to build up staff members and make them feel needed and important.

Hold a staff meeting, express appreciation for the good things the team does, and let them know what changes will need to be made. Take responsibility and apologize for not being assertive enough in holding everybody to this culture, and let them know you will be, going forward.

What advice would you give a dentist that is struggling with case acceptance?

Be concise—Patients don't need to know everything, nor do they want to. Too much information closes their mind to the presented treatment.

Be confident—Especially with specialty procedures, patients can sense any hint of hesitation immediately.

Gain clinical competence—This is for younger dentists like me, but if you are 100% sure you can do a great job and the treatment will benefit the patient, then your presentation will naturally become stronger.

What marketing advice would you give a dentist that is starting out in practice ownership?

Google reviews are king. Challenge yourself to get fifty 5-star reviews as soon as possible. The only way to do this is to establish a system to request them from your patients. You'll be pleased to see the things they write and your staff will feel proud of their work as they see they are part of a great reputation.

What do our dental patients most desire?

Most people want to feel important and they want to be right. Compliment them, make them feel better about themselves. Listen to their desires or fears regarding their dental treatment, and recognize their feelings as valid.

Genuinely express empathy or appreciation. If they feel better about themselves when they are with you, you will have their trust. It's good for relationships and it's good for business.

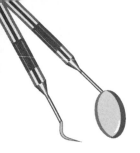

DR. RICK WORKMAN

Founder of Heartland Dental

Justin: *This next interview is with the founder of Heartland Dental, Dr. Rick Workman. There is no doubt Dr. Workman has set himself apart in greatness of achievement with more than 800 dental offices. What he has managed to create is nothing short of incredible, and it does not happen by chance. I've personally never met Dr. Workman—in fact, it wasn't easy to get this interview—but everyone I've talked to that has met him has nothing but glowing things to say about him. I'm happy we were able to include him in this book, because he shares a lot of wisdom in the following interview.*

Dave: *I recall as a Junior in dental school, Dr. Workman and one of his team members bringing us pizza and telling us about their vision for Heartland. It's amazing to see where that vision and his leadership ability have carried him and his company since the early 2000s.*

Background

Rick Workman, DMD, is the founder and executive chairman of Heartland Dental. After many years of practicing full time, Dr. Workman created Heartland Dental, a world-class dental support organization, offering non-clinical, administrative services to supported dentists and team members. Today, Heartland Dental is the largest dental support organization in the nation, with more than 800 supported dental offices in 34 states. Thousands of dentists and team members across the country have taken advantage of the non-clinical support, leading continuing education, and priceless mentorship opportunities available at Heartland Dental to help achieve their goals.

Dr. Workman has over 35 years of experience in the healthcare industry. He is a former president of the Association of Dental Support Organizations (ADSO), a recipient of the Ernst & Young Entrepreneur of the Year Award in their Master's category, the BESI Award (Business Ethics & Social Involvement Award) from the East Central Illinois Development Corporation, and the Richard C. Siemer Outstanding Philanthropist Award from the Southeastern Illinois Community Foundation.

Do you have a favorite success quote or mantra?

There are a few quotes and sayings that have had a strong impact on my career and the success of Heartland Dental. Now these are not my own quotes and have been taken from outside sources, but still have been impactful nonetheless:

"The purpose of education is results producing action."

"Do the right things for the right reasons,
in the right work environment."

"Luck is what happens when
preparation meets opportunity."

In regards to your dental career, what would you like your legacy to be, or how would you like to be remembered?

I would like to be remembered as someone who loved dentistry, and who saw the dentist's responsibility as doing what's best for the patient, understanding what the needs of the patient truly are, and at the same time, learning what it means to be the best dentist possible. And when I say "becoming the best dentist possible," I'm not only referring to providing ideal care. That's a big part of it, but there's so much more involved.

As our profession has transformed (and continues to transform), the realities of practicing have changed. While I was practicing, I saw and experienced firsthand the struggles dentists faced. I spent a career trying to solve the needs for practitioners entering the profession, learning the profession, and surviving the challenges of non-clinical responsibilities. I sought to provide solutions while trying to create systems that created efficiency and quality assurance, which would give patients more access to care and the transparency they deserve. Not all dentists want or need help, but many do. I hopefully helped them and helped changed the profession that had often made them feel "lesser" for desiring or needing that support.

Over the years, I'd like to think I've succeeded in accomplishing many of those things. Heartland Dental has helped countless dentists focus on dentistry, become overall better leaders, and become the dentists they always envisioned becoming. In the process, their patients have benefited. So in answering the question, I want to be remembered as someone who simply wanted to create a better way for dentists so they could provide a higher level of care for patients, who fought to make that vision a reality, and who helped lay a foundation for dentists to receive world-class support for years to come.

What does success mean to you?

I believe success is achieved when any dentist who wants and needs support, is able to receive that support any time they want. No dentist should suffer stress or anxiety because they don't know how to handle non-clinical responsibilities.

In addition, dentists shouldn't feel isolated or alone without being a part of a network of like-minded professionals willing to help without judgement. Dentists would have up-to-date technology and techniques, and practice in state-of-the-art offices staffed by people who are happy, healthy, caring, and competent. If I can help dentists achieve that level of success for themselves, I have succeeded!

What is your biggest fear?

My biggest fear is that while organized dentistry and DSOs grapple over turf, our great profession will be swallowed up by federalized health care or other mass health care systems, basically becoming an afterthought in a public and private national healthcare system. I fear that the myopic focus on dental practice ownership is distracting many from focusing on more pernicious challenges like insurance company mandates, mid-level providers, escalating costs of dental education and establishing a practice, and the practical realities of millennials entering the profession.

Please explain the most challenging time in your career and how you moved past it and thrived on the other side?

There have been several significant learning opportunities in my career. One that comes to mind—when I first realized that my practice in the 1980s had grown beyond my ability to provide all the dentistry, do the business side, and pay the bills. I was in a position where I had to rely on other dentists in our company to make things happen. From that, I began working to solidify our core people in our company. Challenging yes, but it also helped me become better at doctor recruiting, doctor retention, etc. Another challenging time—in the early 2000s, we were forced to realize that being right wasn't always enough. We could be attacked or be vulnerable to attack regardless if we were right or not right. As a company, we had to rely on our faith and principals that if we continue down the path we were going, things would work out in the long run. We were able to move past that by having and nurturing a culture that knew the realities of our organization and had faith in it.

What is your goal-setting process?

This process has expanded over time, but the core element of my process revolves around setting SMART goals. Goals need to be more than sentences on a piece of paper. You have to specifically plan how to achieve your goals. When will you do it and more importantly, why will you do it? Whose support will you need? What will be the end result if successful? What consequences will result if you're not successful? All of these aspects and more need to be considered. By putting your goals into SMART format—specific, measurable, attainable, ROI and timely—you can organize your thoughts into an attainable action plan.

Dave: Typically when I've seen SMART goals discussed, the R stands for realistic. I've always had a hard time with that because BHAGs (Big Hairy Audacious Goals) perhaps would be "unrealistic", but they would also be the most compelling. They really stir emotion and bold action. I so appreciate that Dr. Workman's model has an R that represents Return on Investment.

What is the best investment you have made either inside your career or outside of dentistry?

Two of the best investments we've made at Heartland Dental were NOT acquisitions or equipment investments. They were Walter Hailey's Boot Kamp in the 90s and Bell Leadership over the last decade. From both, we've learned a lot of sage wisdom and the importance of building the right practice and company culture—while most dentists are taught the opposite in school.

These investments have helped us as a company with overcoming struggles, setting the right goals, and creating more powerful communications. In Dr. Bell's Law of Three Voices and also his Law of Three Messages, he explains that the actual words we say only make up 1% of what we communicate. Our tone, body language, and whether the audience trusts and believes that the messenger cares about the audience are much more powerful. Words can lie, but these other aspects are hard to fake.

Looking back, what advice would you give yourself on the day of your dental school graduation?

I would have advised myself to get a mentor and learn that your team is critical to the success of your office. In dental school, dentists are taught that they are the center of the universe in their dental practices, and that everything else more or less orbits around them. Today, I would advise that the team is the center of the universe. Everything orbits around them in terms of office success. While dentists are obviously critical for many aspects of delivering care, their team will ultimately determine the success or failure of their practice. While becoming a great leader can seem daunting at times, being open, positive, and mentally flexible are common attributes of great leaders.

Dave: *"Team is the center of the universe" ... that's worth repeating!*

In your opinion, what separates the top 10% of dentists from the bottom 90%?

Those top 10% are open, positive, and mentally flexible. They have a strong work ethic and self-discipline. They are open to new ideas and techniques, and realize that things will always change. Therefore, they are on a continual journey to grow and achieve excellence. They are confident rather than arrogant, outgoing, and therefore, capable of building relationships easier.

What keeps struggling dentists struggling?

Essentially, because they are the opposite of open, positive, and mentally flexible. They have a victim mentality, and don't understand why the world doesn't accommodate or change around what they want. Where in reality, if you want to succeed, YOU have to adapt to the world around you.

What are the top 3 books every dental practice owner should read?

There are a few I would mention. An oldie but goodie, *How to Win Friends & Influence People* by Dale Carnegie

Megatrends by John Naisbitt made me think about adapting to the future.

The powerful book *The Great Game of Business* by Jack Stack had a big influence.

I also couldn't have succeeded without *Good to Great* by James Collins. It may be the best book since 2000.

If you had to narrow it down to a couple...what traits or skills do you think are most important in running an uncommonly successful practice?

As I mentioned before, being positive is important. Great team members are more likely to follow a positive person than a negative one. You have to have conviction; to have uncommon success, you need uncommon expectations and uncommon goals. You need to take the extra effort. You will have setbacks and disappointments; it's inevitable.

For example, at Heartland Dental, we tend to affiliate with top-10% offices. These doctors have already experienced great success, but when they join us, they still grow. That's because they have that conviction—they're always looking to achieve the next level rather than settle for where they are at.

What is the best business advice you ever received?

I was told, "It's better to copy genius than invent mediocrity." There's so much out there to learn from others who have been in your shoes before and succeeded. Why not learn from their successes and failures rather than starting from scratch and making the same mistakes?

This is where mentorship can be so beneficial. It's also why large DSOs such as Heartland Dental have such an inherent advantage. There is just so much daily sharing of ideas, knowledge, and experiences that solo practitioners have difficulty accessing.

What leadership advice would you give a dentist who has an ineffective culture in their practice?

The key is to gain self-awareness of their strengths and weaknesses. I suggest that they take Bell Leadership with Dr. Bell and also gain 360 anonymous feedback from their team—even if it's difficult to receive, it's feedback that needs to be learned. Ask your team for help and have the courage to listen to them.

Having a mentor is helpful in this situation as well. They can help assess your office culture—what issues are being caused by you and which are being caused by your team. Always remember, a lot of our traits as dentists are a result of our own upbringing, as well as what we learned in dental school. We can't change those experiences, but we can learn that it's never too late to learn how those things affect us. We're not victims. We can get better.

What advice would you give a dentist that is struggling with case acceptance?

Since this is a critical piece in defining whether an office will succeed or struggle, it's extremely important. It's also very complex. It's not as simple as key words or key phrases. There are many other things involved in addition to how you speak to a patient. As I previously mentioned, in Dr. Bell's Law of Three Voices, he describes how body language and tone are even more important than words.

Understanding his Law of Three Messages is also critical. In a dental office, the condition of your office, the technology you have, the dress code of you and your team, and basically the overall atmosphere of your office all send a message. That has to be taken into consideration as well, as that does impact the perception of a patient. Make sure you're representing you and your team to the best of your ability with those external elements.

In regards to communication, be confident and outgoing, but sincere above all. You can get better if you commit to working at it. But recognize that it is a life study, and not a simple skill to master overnight.

What marketing advice would you give a dentist that is starting out in practice ownership?

I would advise to not always believe what you hear, and in your marketing, don't pretend you are something you're not. Be honest with the expectations you set in your marketing. Also, I would advise to seek out a variety of data points from both inside and outside the profession. Outside consultants can also be a great resource for marketing strategy.

It's important to understand that decades ago, many in the industry felt that good dentists didn't need to advertise. I don't think that's the case though; all types of dentists advertise, whether they are good clinicians or not so good. In today's world though, the messages that need to be communicated are different now and perhaps even more important. Patients are more knowledgeable about what they want and have more ways than ever to access those things.

Whether they're looking for a family dentist, cosmetic dentistry, pediatric dentistry, practices with high levels of technology, etc. With what your office is and what your culture is, think about how you can best communicate that to patients honestly.

What do our dental patients most desire?

This may be a cliché, but patients look for integrity in their dentist or dental office. They want to know whether you truly care about them and their needs. They will make more judgments on whether you really care about them rather than the words they hear from you or the equipment you own.

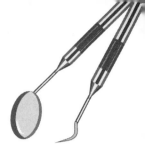

DR. WADE PILLING

Aesthetic Smiles

Justin: *This next interviewee was the first person I started following on DentalTown many years ago. I've always enjoyed Wade's take on life and specifically investments outside of hands-on dentistry. I've consulted with him on several investments, and appreciate his willingness to always lend his expertise.*

Background

I was born and raised in Alberta, Canada. Grew up loving the outdoors. Skiing, backpacking, adventures. Still do. Currently live in Eagle, Idaho and practice full-time dentistry focusing on cosmetic, implant, and reconstructive dentistry. I also lecture about clinical dentistry.

I've owned multiple practices in my career. I also invest in other businesses like hotels, real estate, car washes, and other diversified businesses as a form of passive income.

Most importantly, I live life to the fullest. I have a wife and 6 kids. We travel and play like no one else. I make sure to take 10–12 weeks of vacation each year to explore and have adventures with my family. My wife and I are also spartan racers. We travel the country competing in obstacle course racing. Work hard, play hard is our motto.

Please explain your style of practice (practice size, location, procedure mix, etc.)

My current practice consists of me and a partner, and our location is in the Boise, Idaho area. Our practice style is a one-stop shop for most procedures. Between the two of us, our skill set is able to address most of our patients' needs. My part of the practice is heavy into elective procedures. Smile makeovers, full mouth rehabs, ortho, and implants are the bulk of my procedures.

We still have a general dentistry side of our practice, but many seek us out for these elective smile-enhancing procedures, as that is where my training and skill set is best utilized. It makes for a low-volume style of practice, which I love. Not the only way to practice, but it is a good way to practice. We have invested heavily in technology such as CBCT, 3D, Cad Cam, 3D printing, guided surgery, etc. It creates a fun way to practice and gives us more predictable results.

Do you have a favorite success quote or mantra?

"There are no strangers on the course today.
There are only teammates you have not met yet."

People think true capitalism and success means winners and losers. Trample the weak and hurdle the dead to get to your goals. But when you treat those you work with, and patients, clients, etc. as teammates all working towards a common goal, and you just playing a role in helping them—you'll find success, but also joy in the journey and the way you obtained your success. I prefer to treat everyone I work with as a teammate and I am their advocate to help them succeed. I don't look at relationships as something I can milk or profit from. No one is seen as a profit center for me.

In regards to your dental career, what would you like your legacy to be, or how would you like to be remembered?

I want my legacy to be one of excellence and honesty. I want my patients to know I had a commitment to excellence every time I worked on them, and that I did my best.

What does success mean to you?

I can do what I want when I want. I can steer my life the way I want. Not held back by any pressures whether they be financial, social, etc. I control my life. I can donate when I want, help when I want, have fun when I want, provide when I want. Freedom, essentially.

What is your morning routine (first 1–2 hrs of the day)?

Wake up at 5:00am. Go hit the gym for at least an hour. Throw heavy stuff around, let out some of the beast inside. Start the day crushing stuff. I don't drink coffee, so the adrenaline and endorphin rush is what gets me motivated for the day.

What is your biggest fear?

Letting my family down. Not just financially really, but as a parent and spouse. Not living up to my duties and promises to watch out and care and lead and encourage them. Letting them down would be worse than any financial mistake I could ever make. Priorities. I realize money is only money. It can be rebuilt or remade or earned. You can't take it with you.

Please explain the most challenging time in your career and how you moved past it and thrived on the other side?

The most challenging part of my career was when I first graduated. I built a brand-new office building that was 9000 square feet. Half for me and half to rent out. My goal was to have a tenant pay my mortgage. I built a beautiful office in an expensive building. I worked as an associate while my office was being built. I ended up leaving that position because something didn't feel right.

So now at 1 year out of school, I was about 2 million dollars in debt and had no patients. I also had a building that sat empty for 5 years because I couldn't find renters. And when I did, they bolted after 2 months of rent—after I had spent $175,000 on TI's for them. I had to start digging out of that hole.

I had no business sense on how to run a practice. No savvy ideas. My goal was to treat people right and do good dentistry, and hopefully there would be money left over to pay the bills and myself. That was my goal. To treat people right and ignore the fact I had such huge debt. Rather than stress out about the debt, I put it out of my mind.

I treated patients right, I invested in lots of CE to provide more services, and it all worked out fine. I didn't let debt crush me. I focused on my goals. I bought 2 other practices during the next 5 years and flipped them. I looked for opportunities that made sense.

What is your goal-setting process?

I'm a big picture guy. I don't do things on a micro level. Some people need to. But I keep a big picture and let the rest fall into place as it will. I plan my goals around what I want to do in my life and then mold the practice or businesses around that. If an investment is going to interfere with some of those goals, I pass on it.

What is the best investment you have made either inside your career or outside of dentistry?

Best investment inside my career was taking the necessary training to be able to give my patients what they were asking for. Whether it's ortho, veneers, implants, gum grafting, botox, or general dentistry. Being able to confidently take care of your patients has turned our practice into an efficient machine that can closely control the outcomes. Outside of dentistry, my best investments have come through starting early and investing in low-cost index funds through tax advantaged vehicles such as Roths, backdoor Roths, or 401Ks. This is and should always be your primary vehicle before turning to other, more diversified investments.

Looking back, what advice would you give yourself on the day of your dental school graduation?

Grow your practice by growing your skill set. Don't be afraid to learn, no matter the cost and time away from your practice. Your practice will always be your primary vehicle to fund your investments and lifestyle and goals or hobbies. Don't be distracted by stuff outside of your practice until you've built a well-oiled machine. Know what your patients want and give it to them.

Dave: Great advice. It's easy to see the "costs" of CE: tuition, loss of income, hotel, flights, etc. But if you can do a decent job with selecting good CE and implementing, a weekend course can pay dividends for the rest of your career.

In your opinion, what separates the top 10% of dentists from the bottom 90%?

Confidence. The upper 10% feel confident in presenting treatment and evaluating people. They understand how to care about their patients and understand what they want. People buy from people they like. The top 10% know how to listen, know how to care, and know how to relate and give patients what they want without being pushy. They know how to be the patient's advocate in getting them to their goals.

What keeps struggling dentists struggling?

They aren't great communicators, or they haven't surrounded themselves with great communicators. A confused or unconvinced patient will never accept treatment. There are some amazing doctors out there that just can't communicate. And if they can't, they don't have teams that can either. Someone needs to be able to communicate the value of treatment to the patients. We need to start being interested in our patients and make sure they know we are.

What are the top 3 books every dental practice owner should read?

Bonded Porcelain Restorations: A Clinical Guide to What Excellence Looks Like by Pascal Magne. After reading it, you should be able to recognize excellence and be inspired to do it yourself.

The 7 Habits of Highly Effective People by Steven R. Covey. I know everyone knows this book, but it really is simple stuff to becoming an effective person.

The Only Guide to a Winning Investment Strategy You'll Ever Need by Larry Swedroe.

If you had to narrow it down to a couple...what traits or skills do you think are most important in running an uncommonly successful practice?

Ability to motivate employees. Being positive, finding what they are good at, and setting them up for success. A winning team is important.

What is a skill or procedure you've added since graduating from dental school that has had a major positive impact on your practice?

Orthodontics.

What is the best business advice you ever received?

Increased production/collections will take care of your overhead problem.

What leadership advice would you give a dentist who has an ineffective culture in their practice?

Compliment your staff when they do something right. Too much negativity will bring the office morale down.

Justin: I preach this as well with my clients. Compliment your staff whenever you get the chance! It's the quickest way to increase the behaviors you want to see your team exhibit, and it builds their confidence. If they don't know what to do or how to act in the first place, train them well, then compliment the effort and behavior along the way.

What advice would you give a dentist that is struggling with case acceptance?

Don't act desperate. Tell the patient this is the best you can do for them and whenever they are ready, you're here to help them. Don't scare patients. Tell them what can happen, but always remember you're here to help the patient first, and sometimes that is on their schedule. Give people options. Let them know they can stay in your practice getting maintenance work until they are ready to do comprehensive treatment. Don't pressure, don't chase away. Remember you are their advocate here.

What marketing advice would you give a dentist that is starting out in practice ownership?

Ask your patients for referrals. It only seems hard on the surface. Get the staff doing it as well. It really takes nothing at all to say, "Thanks for letting us care for you. If you have any friends or family that are as awesome as you, we'd love to help them have a great experience too."

What do our dental patients most desire?

Health. Whatever their definition of health is, that's what they want. It could be pain free, functioning, looks, or all of the above.

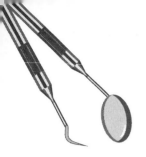

DR. PETER THOMPSON

Thompson Smiles

Justin: *I met Peter at a PDA event in 2016. His is a story I love and one that intrigued me right away. You may or may not have known his name up until now, but he has built a tremendous private practice in rural Eastern New Mexico, and we felt he absolutely fit the criteria of what we were looking for in this book.*

Background

Dentistry has allowed me to change so many lives for the better, and that is what I cherish about this profession. I am an avid pilot, golfer, skier, and husband of 23 years and father of 3 children.

Please explain your style of practice (practice size, location, procedure mix, etc.)

I live in a rural community in Eastern New Mexico, isolated in nature, and there's about 17,000 in our local community. I produce $2.7 million annually on 3–4 days a week with about 6–8 weeks off a year.

Do you have a favorite success quote or mantra?

You don't know what you don't know until you learn what you don't know.

In regards to your dental career, what would you like your legacy to be, or how would you like to be remembered?

I just want the people in my community and state to appreciate the positive changes we've made in their lives.

What does success mean to you?

Having the freedom to pursue things you love doing.

What is your morning routine (first 1–2 hrs of the day)?

Up at 4:45, cardio for 30 minutes, and then workout for 1 hour... shower at the office and hit it‼

What is your biggest fear?

Crazy roller coasters.

Please explain the most challenging time in your career and how you moved past it and thrived on the other side?

After 2 years of practice, just frustrated with insurance companies and the mentality they bring, we went fee for service with the exception of one insurance company...now we are 90% fee for service.

What is your goal-setting process?

Visualize, verbalize, take baby steps every day!

Dave: If you don't have a strong visualization practice and are interested in implementing one, check out DreamItAlive.com. It makes the powerful process very easy.

What is the best investment you have made either inside your career or outside of dentistry?

Continuing education.

Looking back, what advice would you give yourself on the day of your dental school graduation?

Realize...you know just enough to hurt people. Start taking GOOD CE. Learn technology, learn occlusion, learn implants well, learn to treatment plan. Live very modestly and invest in yourself and your continuing education.

In your opinion, what separates the top 10% of dentists from the bottom 90%?

Comprehensive treatment planning and verbal skills.

What keeps struggling dentists struggling?

Narrow vision and a crippling fear of the unknown.

Dave: There have been a few points in my career that I felt stuck. In hindsight, my issues were exactly as Peter mentioned: being myopic and scared to take a critical next step.

If you had to narrow it down to a couple...what traits or skills do you think are most important in running an uncommonly successful practice?

Vision and confidence in yourself.

What is a skill or procedure you've added since graduating from dental school that has had a major positive impact on your practice?

IV sedation, implants, cerec, occlusion, and smile design.   '

What is the best business advice you ever received?

Live modestly and invest in your practice and yourself.

What leadership advice would you give a dentist who has an ineffective culture in their practice?

Seek help!!

What advice would you give a dentist that is struggling with case acceptance?

Seek help!!

What do our dental patients most desire?

Affordable options.

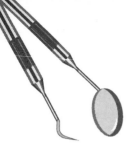

DR. STEVEN L. RASNER

DMD, MAGD – Pearl Smiles

Background

In 1981, Owens-Illinois—the 6th largest glass plant in the world—closed its doors. What followed was a domino effect of failed businesses, staggering unemployment, and a devastatingly bleak economy. That was the year after Dr. Steven Rasner opened his practice in the same town. Regrettably, since that time, Bridgeton, NJ has remained nationally ranked for its unemployment, poverty level, and lack of growth.

During this same period, Dr. Rasner has nurtured a private, fee-for-service practice that commands fees in the top percentile in the nation. It grosses over $4.1 million per year on a 4-day work-week with a "2 day per week" associate and a "substantial bottom line." His team of 16 has been with the practice an average of 16 years. Dr. Rasner takes an active role in his community and received a Congressional Recognition Award in 2000 for his civic contributions.

Dr. Rasner has published multiple books, including: *The Protocol Book*; *The Art of Getting Paid*; and *The Bullet Proof Guide to the Extraordinary Practice*.

Dave: Steve is one of the most powerful speakers I've ever seen on a dental conference stage (and I've seen a lot of them). If you ever see him on the schedule at a conference, do yourself the favor of going to his class.

What does success mean to you?

Success is living your life unequivocally on your terms. Specifically, working when you want to work and not working when you choose to be off. Because you can. Don't underestimate this seemingly mundane expression. Your career and life are going to fly by more quickly than you would like.

Trust me on this: most of your colleagues will live their lives on the terms of their bank loans, not their true wishes. Why? Because most people (and dentists are just people) can't resist the urge to reward themselves with the car and the house, then the shore house. Not to mention private schools and first class everything. And most dentists simply don't make enough to sustain that life style. Doing what you want when you are in your thirties and forties only matters if you can live life on your own terms in the latter stages of your career.

I have given presentations for 20 years and have met literally thousands of dentists. Unless someone gifted it you, the common denominator of older successful professionals is that they conserved early in their careers. They had a modest house and a 6-year-old car. They had low credit card debt and high credit scores. They paid with cash or put significant money down.

They resisted the universal bad investments like a new boat or car or time shares. And they benefited from the power of compounding interest or early capital accumulations. You know what else? They get to take off 6 weeks per year. They get to spend 10 days off when they visit their first grandchild or attend one of many weddings you will attend when you are in your 50s and 60s. What they don't do is orchestrate their lives around 3 days off here, 4 days off there because they are not free.

If you really want freedom, then you have to start early and be willing to say not yet.

Please explain the most challenging time in your career and how you moved past it and thrived on the other side?

I hesitated to answer this one because I never wanted it be my legacy; but it is just too good of an ultimate answer to not include it. It is for one of you out there right now with your own story developing that perhaps no one knows about other than your inner circle. Maybe it's a health issue. Maybe it's financial doom. If one day you find your back against the wall and can't take one more bad day, then perhaps you can draw from this and find your way back to success.

Life is long and we all go through stuff. I had life-threatening lung cancer at 54 (Stage 3 non-small cell adenocarcinoma); crippling back fusions 5 years after the bout with cancer. I lost my son when he was 22 and I'll never get over that, but none of those turn a community against you. People naturally sympathize and cheer you back to life.

Let me tell you what isn't the same: a federal indictment at 32 years old because you somehow were mixed up in the largest cocaine ring ever uncovered in the Northeastern United States. Let me begin by stating it was my own fault; no one held a gun to my head and made me purchase an illegal drug. I knew it was wrong, and I did it anyway.

In fairness to me, the circumstances were at best bizarre. Back then, as a senior in dental school, you are assigned a junior (who hasn't really worked on patients yet) and help them transition into the clinical practice of dentistry. You don't choose them; the school does. Well, my junior partner was a great guy; it seemed that everyone knew him and liked him. He was a likable guy with one problem. He was an intricate part of an existing cocaine ring, already in full operation, run by 5 dental students. I said dental students! On my life, I was never aware of any of this until December of my senior year. I wasn't the drug-taking kind of kid. Sounds like movie material, right? Well, it's the subject of 2 books and several television documentaries. Although I had nothing to do with the operations, I did continue to buy until I was indicted 2 years out of dental school.

Good Morning America kind of news: coast to coast. A hundred and ten "yuppies", as in doctors, lawyers, stock brokers charged. But as the dominos fell, I was one of the first thirteen and no one knows your true role. And it doesn't matter. Outside of child molestation, it was the single most career-ending act a professional could have committed.

Front page news. In the end, I was charged with buying a controlled substance over the telephone. I was sentenced to 5 years probation, 10 months in a halfway house, and enormous fines. At 32, I had a 10 month old, was $400,000 in debt (fines and attorney fees) and here is where you really begin to lose hope: my license was revoked to ever practice again. As in ever.

Now what was the original question? Oh yeah, a most challenging time. Listen, I caused it all, but that didn't take the pain out of the sheer embarrassment I brought my family, my university, and my profession. For the next 2 years, I basically hid from the world. I would take courses in nearby states, sit in the back with sunglasses on, hoping no one would notice me. I sold vacuum cleaners to keep a roof over my head. Let me tell you one more thing: God forbid you ever face such obstacles, but when you do, it isn't just your friends that disappear. People have their own lives and own problems to deal with, and you find yourself very much on your own.

So how the did I get to today?

I know you have likely heard it through this book, but I never quit. I loved being a dentist. The short 2 years I practiced before this came down gave me a glimpse of what my future might be like. Patients came to me in droves, and although I was pretty raw, it felt like I could one day be really good. I wouldn't give it up. After the board of dentistry hung up on me after many weeks of calls, I just put my

2-year-old in the car with my wife one day and drove 2 hours to Newark, New Jersey. On the way, my son somehow poked his eye, resulting in a scratched cornea, so my first stop was the ER.

Didn't stop me. I took the elevator to the floor of the dental board and was met by a not-so-friendly representative. He literally blocked the door's path with his arm and said, "I told you; we are very busy." Maybe it was the desperation in my eyes or my screaming 2-year-old, but he conceded to give me "5 minutes and not a second more!"

Forty-five minutes later, I had a verbal promise to be on a board schedule. I had hope. I had been out of the practice 2 years. My father had come out of retirement to try to hold down the fort, but I wasn't even allowed on the property. I had maxed all my credit cards, I was behind in any due payments, and no one would dream of lending me money. Any good will had expired.

Ten days before my hearing, my father died of a stroke at the practice, while covering for me. Try carrying that around for the past 30 years. You can conjecture all you want about this or that, but it sure feels like I had something to do with that outcome. Now the practice was literally closed. My lawyer had no expectations for me. Even though I was on the docket, we weren't sure the board would get to my appeal.

Unbeknownst to me, a powerful New Jersey politician and dear friend of my father would make a call to the board to try to help me. After the hearing, he would tell me that they felt badly about my plight, but I wasn't getting my license back. Not now. Maybe never. In August of 1985, I walked out of the hearing with my license. Not 6 weeks later at the next board meeting—but that day. I asked them that if they felt any inclination to help me, I needed the help today. Not tomorrow. I told them I would never let them down. That the only thing they would ever hear associated with my name would be positive and good for the profession.

As of this writing, I have given over 250 presentations over 20 years. I have been on the cover of *Dentistry Today* as one of the top educators

12 years running. It would have been easy to run from South Jersey and open up where no one knew me. I never left. I'm sure I am not everyone's cup of tea, but overall I have put together a practice both clinically and business-wise that would be the envy of many.

I have given back to all segments of the community from law enforcement to the mentally challenged. I have been honored by my community and received a United States congressional award in 2001 for years of community service. I never gave up. I didn't waste time feeling sorry for myself. No matter how many times I was told no, I made another call or wrote another letter. I owned the problem. I never blamed anyone other than myself. I fought to this day to regain my integrity. My reputation. I did the right thing whether someone was watching me or not. And I never ever took the privilege of a license for granted again.

Two years ago, I appeared once again before the New Jersey Board of Dentistry. I wasn't in trouble. I requested permission to run a course from my office where doctors can come in from anywhere in the US without a NJ license and learn live hands-on atraumatic extractions.

There aren't many places like this in the U.S., let alone New Jersey. It was a huge request.

My next class this Spring is once again sold out. Never quit. You hear me?

Dave: *Dr. Rasner told this story on the* Relentless Dentist Podcast. *I still remember the chills I had as he told it. Many of us have had our challenges in the profession. But it's hard to imagine starting out a career with the dental world seemingly against you and battling back to reach the pinnacle of dental success.*

Justin: *There have been several times in this book where Dave and I have needed to edit things down a bit, but this story was too powerful to edit. There were many things that stood out to me in Dr. Rasner's story, but I truly respect the fact that he owned his problem. He didn't shift the blame. The words "It was my fault" are often avoided at all costs in our lives, but often they're where true change begins.*

In your opinion, what separates the top 10% of dentists from the bottom 90%?

The number one factor that separates the very best is a visceral gut desire. It is that simple.

There is a popular video out there on a motivational circuit, by Eric Thomas. He describes a story about a young man who wanted success. He wanted to be on the same level of the guru he sought advice from. The guru said, "Fine, meet me tomorrow morning on the beach." At 4:00 am the next morning, the young man was ready, dressed immaculately in a suit. The guru asked him, "How bad do you want it?" "Really bad," he replied. So he grabbed his hand and began walking toward the water. By the time he was waist deep, the young man is thinking, this guy is crazy; I didn't ask to be a lifeguard. By the time the water was at the level of his mouth, the young man became hesitant. When you adopt the attitude "I will do whatever it takes" and you mean it. The guru asked again, "How bad do you want it?" As he walked a bit further, the guru held his head under the water. As he was about to pass out, he let him up and said, "When you want to be successful as badly as you want to breathe (when you can't), then you will be successful!"

When you don't care about what's on TV; when you don't care about partying, sleeping in late, or staying later for a potential new case, or working at night or Saturday. When you adopt the attitude that you will do whatever it takes early in your career; when you get back up after the setbacks you will face; when you go back to your desk and write out a new ad campaign because the last one fell flat; when you write a brand new ad because the last 3 didn't draw the right front desk receptionist; when you don't waste time sulking or feeling sorry for yourself because you are not there yet: That is a gut desire that few individuals in any walk of life can honestly state they own. The top 10% just outworked everyone else and refused to give in to the many obstacles we all face.

Justin: Eric Thomas is one of, if not my most, favorite motivational speaker. Literally everyday I drove into my office, I would listen to his talks. Day after day after day. It helped me prepare my mind for the day at the office.

If you had to narrow it down to a couple...what traits or skills do you think are most important in running an uncommonly successful practice?

The number one trait is continually communicating to the team what you as the boss feel is important.

Remember this: No one is going to benefit from the success more or fall harder from the failure of your practice than you. You have the most to gain and the most to lose. So because of this axiom, you must continue to lead. This translates into reminder emails going out first thing Monday morning, reminding different departments that you want them to re-implement protocols that you installed a month ago. For example, going hygiene through schedules of that week and notating all patients with a history of RP & SC; or doing a better job of charting abfractions and recessions and documenting with photographs.

Perhaps you will remind the front desk team about getting copies of driver licenses or cell phone numbers and email contact updates. It doesn't matter what it is; it will often seem overwhelming that you the boss have to continually remind the team of what is important. Super successful offices have systems that don't end up in the closet 3 months after they started because you simply didn't allow it! The good news is that if you hang in there, eventually new ideas become habit.

Justin: How many of us have made great declarations in our office, only to see them completed well for a week and disappear completely within a month? Repetition is what makes something a habit. You have to stay on your team until the habits you want to see become ingrained as second nature, or real lasting change will not happen.

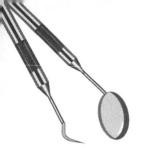

DR. PETER BOULDEN

Atlanta Dental Spa,
Bulletproof Dentist Podcast

Background

A native Atlantan, I'm a 41 year old father of 3, and husband of 1. Have 4 dental locations under 2 brands. Currently under contract with another practice. Love dentistry and the business of dentistry. Fanatic fan of technology and scale. I'm a 10x thinker to a fault.

Please explain your style of practice (practice size, location, procedure mix, etc.)

Three FFS practices. 1 PPO/FFS mix. Revenues north of $6.5MM/year. Focus on comprehensive dentistry, implant, and cosmetic dentistry in the practice. We have 7 doctors and 10 hygienists.

Practices focus on high-end dentistry and high-end customer experience.

Do you have a favorite success quote or mantra?

> *"It is not the critic who counts; not the man who points out*
> *how the strong man stumbles, or where the doer of deeds*

could have done them better. The credit belongs to the man
who is actually in the arena, whose face is marred by dust
and sweat and blood; who strives valiantly; who errs, who
comes short again and again, because there is no effort
without error and shortcoming; but who does actually strive
to do the deeds; who knows great enthusiasms, the great
devotions; who spends himself in a worthy cause; who at
the best knows in the end the triumph of high achievement,
and who at the worst, if he fails, at least fails while daring
greatly, so that his place shall never be with those cold
and timid souls who neither know victory nor defeat."

—THEODORE ROOSEVELT

Let me explain why this is my favorite quote, because it doesn't exactly ROLL off the tongue. This quote reminds me to "get in the game of life". Don't be afraid to fail, don't question your success, and sure as shit don't listen to naysayers.

In regards to your dental career, what would you like your legacy to be, or how would you like to be remembered?

Honestly, the only people I care about how I'm remembered are my family, my friends, and my teams. Beyond that, I really don't care. But amongst them, I would hope that I was remembered for bringing value to their life. My existence in their life made their life a bit better.

What does success mean to you?

Success means being able to do what I want, with who I want, when I want. Success is all about freedom.

What is your morning routine (first 1–2 hrs of the day)?

5 minutes of prayer

5 minutes of gratitude (it's the antidote for fear, depression, unhappiness, etc.)

5 minutes of betterment (TED talk, youtube video, article)

5 minutes of filling out "wheel of balance" (my own developed balance chart)

What is your biggest fear?

Being old and having regret. Then not having the time or energy to fix it.

Please explain the most challenging time in your career and how you moved past it and thrived on the other side?

WORST YEAR 2015—A 10-year partnership in my practice dissolved, and I spent my life savings to keep the practice. So essentially I was wiped out financially. A month later, discovered that I had been embezzled from for over $535K. My son was born 6 weeks premature. I wanted to be fully engaged with my family for him, but I couldn't, because life was falling around me. 2015 was also when I had the highest clinical demands on me and my biggest production year ever. One would think this was awesome, but I was truly at the end of my rope—physically & emotionally. I was burnt out and literally had to pep talk myself on the end of my bed each morning to, "DON'T QUIT, DON'T GIVE UP because so many people depend on you."

BEST YEAR 2016—I kept telling myself in 2015, "Don't quit." One more day. Let's just finish the year and then re-calibrate. Life was kicking my ass and I knew it was unsustainable. If I could just make it to the Christmas break, it would allow me time to re-engineer my life. I knew I HAD to be intentional about designing my life, starting in 2016, instead of the random forces being in control. I cut back on my clinical calendar—going from 16 days a month to 9 days a month. I hired an Executive Assistant to really help me accomplish more and not be overwhelmed with the operations of it all...this was one of the best things I ever did, even though I questioned whether I could "justify" it. I basically reverse engineered what I wanted my life to look like—personally, professionally.

What is your goal-setting process?

It's constant. I'm a raving fan. Mine are reviewed daily...sometimes multiple times daily. I set goals for a month and a year. Three- and five-year goals are bullshit because we live in such dynamic times. I look at my modest goals and make myself say what would happen if these were 10x'd.

What is the best investment you have made either inside your career or outside of dentistry?

I can't point to a SINGLE best investment. Honestly, I have 6 pieces of real estate that have worked well. My practice could be considered the best investment. I DO NOT invest in things that I cannot control—the stock market, mutual funds, silent/angel investing, etc. I have NOT gotten involved in some new business ventures, because I couldn't be in control.

My best investment advice is ALWAYS invest in yourself, double and triple down on your strengths and passions, AND most important, stay in your damn lane (meaning just because you have run a great dental practice, don't think that uniquely qualifies you to open a Subway or Smoothie shop, for example).

Lastly, don't forget that investing in people in your life is the MOST fulfilling. There are likely people supporting your dream, goal, vision, etc. Make sure to support them reciprocally on personal development and also their goals and dreams.

Looking back, what advice would you give yourself on the day of your dental school graduation?

Congrats, let's grab a beer and let me explain how now the hard work begins. You're not entitled to anything just because you have a diploma. If you want it, you have to create it. Dreams are FREE, but the HUSTLE is sold separately.

Dave: I love this perspective. Every high-performing dentist that I've ever had a deep conversation with realizes that a dental license is only the ticket to enter the game. Most see it as a "golden ticket" that gives them unlimited opportunity, should they have the courage and ambition to aggressively pursue their professional goals.

In your opinion, what separates the top 10% of dentists from the bottom 90%?

People skills. Being able to lead emphatically. Being able to present treatment emphatically. Never letting people confuse your kindness for weakness.

Vision. Most of the top-10% dentists created their own navigation/GPS a long time ago. They knew where they wanted to go, the practice they wanted to create, etc. Just setting off with your fingers crossed and a "hope it goes well" is a crazy proposition to me.

What keeps struggling dentists struggling?

They're not in control of their environment. They have a "people-dependent" practice, not a systems-dependent practice. They've had trouble delegating & feel they're always the best person for every job and thus never move past the "glorified job" stage. This struggle leads to burnout.

Dave: I get lots of Relentless Dentist listener emails. Many of them are from dentists who are struggling. At the core of that struggle is what Peter mentions here: being "out of control". I usually have to politely point out that they are in denial. They are in denial that leadership is their #1 responsibility, that they need to have a grasp on their practice numbers, and that they need to engineer systems within their practice. It's natural to want to focus on clinical dentistry. But the only true way to be in control is to embrace the many hats we wear as practice owners.

What are the top 3 books every dental practice owner should read?

Built to Sell by John Warrillow
The Magic of Thinking Big by David J. Schwartz
The Ultimate Sales Machine by Chet Holmes

If you had to narrow it down to a couple...what traits or skills do you think are most important in running an uncommonly successful practice?

Situational and self awareness: Being aware of your practice environment from a macro scale all the way to the micro. It's only when you humbly acknowledge something needs fixing that change can occur. That's where situational and self awareness start to blend. When you fly planes, pilots are taught to constantly scan the sky and be "situationally aware" of their surroundings...and they should NOT have their head down looking at the instruments, checklists, or controls constantly. Fly the plane (practice)!

Fear of failure: So many people are paralyzed by "what if". "What if I invest in this new office and I can't afford it?" "What if I do this marketing and I don't get XXX ROI?" What if, what if, what if. Whether you think you can or you can't, you're right. In my opinion, I see a lot of scarcity mentality in dentistry as a whole, not the abundant thinking they deserve to have.

What is a skill or procedure you've added since graduating from dental school that has had a major positive impact on your practice?

Clinically, I dove DEEP into cosmetic dentistry and got a name for it in my city.

On the business side, once I graduated, I become a student of marketing, branding, and systems. Read tons of books on customer service.

I'm still learning more about both daily, and hope to keep learning every day, because if I feel like I have NOTHING TO LEARN, I'm going to stop doing dentistry.

What is the best business advice you ever received?

My Dad (and likely his Dad) always said, "If it were easy, everyone could do it." This applies to so many things in life.

What leadership advice would you give a dentist who has an ineffective culture in their practice?

The leader is responsible for ineffective culture. It may be because you created a vacuum (lack of culture) which allowed someone to fill in with "bad" culture. Or simply, the culture you set out to create is ineffective or inauthentic. Either way you need to have EXTREME ACCOUNTABILITY, which ironically, would be a great step for creating an effective culture.

What advice would you give a dentist that is struggling with case acceptance?

Find out where you are...literally video record yourself. Look at your tone and your body language. Are you being perceptive to where THEY (patients) are in the dental process?

People give tells when they're excited, confident, scared, or confused. It's your job to pick up on that and modify your treatment presentation, verbiage, tonality, and body language. EQ is so much more important than IQ.

Oh, and we get it, you're smart, but stop talking like an engineer, because no one likes that.

What marketing advice would you give a dentist that is starting out in practice ownership?

Get on YouTube and start learning. In today's era, you'll be hard pressed to NOT be able to find copious information on any skill you're trying to develop or learn. The content is there, but our desire has to be commensurate.

There is NO excuse for you NOT to be a master marketer. Remember that you're not just someone in a technical job, but you're running a technical business. Just because you have a high technical skill does not uniquely qualify you to run that technical business. You must learn that.

Create systems until you feel like a robot. Constantly audit where you are and "what's next?" Remember that you have MANY who depend on you...and likely those people have people who are dependent on them. Don't take this lightly. Hustle, plan, and lead like a lot of people's livelihoods depend on your actions and decisions... because they do!

What do our dental patients most desire?

The same thing all people do. Value. Value in relationship. Value in getting out of pain. Value in being able to smile now. Value in a "different" dental experience than they had as a kid. Focus on giving value to others and your practice will grow.

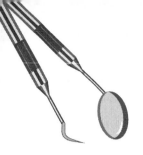

DR. SCOTT LEUNE

Founder and CEO
of Breakaway Practice

Dave: I attended Scott's Breakaway Seminar when it was still held in a small hotel room in San Antonio, a few months before I opened my practice in 2009. We relied heavily on the systems we learned that weekend and saved thousands on the equipment and buildout, due to the advice we got from Scott. This is a CE course I'm constantly recommending both new and seasoned practice owners attend.

Justin: *I've gotten to talk to Scott a few times now, and I think most would agree that operating dental practices is definitely in his "genius zone". Scott's systematic approach to running practices has made Breakaway a wonderful resource for dentists all over the world.*

Background

Dr. Leune graduated from UT Health Science Center School of Dentistry in 2005. His dental career began with 3 startup practices in San Antonio, which grew to 80 staff, 10 dentists, and a call center in a very short time.

These practices continued to average a combined total of over 700 new patients per month and were all managed by Dr. Leune working a mere 4 days per month. In 2011, Dr. Leune started 7 practices in the Dallas-Fort Worth area, opening them within a 2-month timespan. Over the last 4 years, through Breakaway's Consulting Program, Dr. Leune has helped build approximately 100 startup practices nationwide. He has recently merged his Breakaway Companies and partners with other entrepreneurs to form Dental Whale, a company focused on elevating private dentists to be on an even playing field with the corporate groups in dentistry.

Please explain your style of practice (practice size, location, procedure mix, etc.)

Location: San Antonio (home office), Nationwide (dental practices). I have owned 11 startups in the past, I have consulted dentists in another 100+ startups, we have 17,000 dentists we support through our services, and we help manage the operations of 1,000 practices today.

Team size: Approximately 150 employees at the home office, and around 850 employees nationwide.

If you had to narrow it down to a couple...what traits or skills do you think are most important in running an uncommonly successful practice?

Breakaway Practice has four main focuses:

1 Innovation – doing this in a new, disruptive, smarter way.

2 Growth – making sure everything we do helps private dental practices grow.

3 Service – giving elevated levels of reporting, customer service meetings, and general help.

4 Accuracy – auditing heavily to ensure the highest level of accuracy we can attain.

In a dental office, I believe the four main drivers of growth are:

1   Patient Flow – this includes new patient attraction and the retention of existing patients. Many factors affect these items, including marketing, phone answer rate, appointment conversion rate, reappointment rates, and more.

2   Diagnosis – high performing practices will typically diagnose 4x what they produce. To increase the amount of dentistry we diagnose, we focus mainly on two items: a) Learning new procedures and b) Implementing a disciplined system for ensuring we comprehensively diagnose every patient. I have noticed that it is common for us busy dentists in the heat of our daily battle to cut corners on diagnosis and speed up our exam times. Creating a disciplined, systematic approach helps counteract our own tendencies.

3   Case Acceptance – there are many factors to increasing case acceptance, including what the hygienist says, what the dentist says, what we show the patient, what the treatment coordinator says, what our payment options are, as well as outside factors such as how they heard about us or what type of marketing they responded to. All of these things are changeable and have "best practices" ways of maximizing acceptance.

4   Managing our schedule capacity properly – just because we grow patient flow, diagnose fully, and get higher case acceptance doesn't mean we actually do more dentistry. We must manage our capacity properly and expand as soon as the practice asks us to. Doing this is extremely important in a growing practice, but must be done in a healthy and balanced way so that we reduce our costs and risks of expansion.

Of course, these drivers must exist in an environment where we have excellent clinical quality, excellent patient/customer service, and a disciplined, healthy cost structure of performing the care and managing the operations.

How do you maintain your level of success?

I feel success is derived much from what our small daily habits are. Are we auditing every day? Do we have the proper habits set up to reach our goals? Are we saying the perfect thing on the phone? Are we saying the perfect thing in the op? How does our office look, smell, feel, sound, act? These are all habits we create. These are the practices we perform, and I want to make sure these are Best Practices. It is vital, in my opinion, that we create a checklist of habits (best practices) to perform every day, week, and month. Determine the core drivers of our success and put those into a checklist of habits so that we are motivated to complete them. It's about the small frequent steps we take...not the singular large one.

Is there anything you do on a daily (or close to daily) basis that keeps you motivated?

I measure what I want to improve. Forcing myself to measure it every day keeps me motivated to win at that number. If I find myself losing motivation, I pay someone to coach me and keep me going.

What do you do or listen to on your way to work?

I listen to loud Christian Music on Satellite Radio in my jeep with the doors off. I love starting the day in a good mood with free-flowing air, listening to music. Positivity is an important part of seeing opportunity and managing challenges.

How do you deal with an underperforming team member in the office?

The key is actually recognizing it early enough...I do that through tracking some core numbers which tell me how the performance is going of every team member. Once I recognize a problem, I attempt to train them and retrain them. I then follow up with immediate and frequent auditing. If I still can't influence change, I issue a written warning. Eventually, I terminate them (usually to the happiness of everyone else who was having to do their job for them). The better a leader I am, the less chance I need to terminate someone.

Statistics say only a small % of dentists are financially prepared to retire at age 65. Why do you think that is?

We have delayed gratification financially as we attempt to get through a lot of school, take on a lot of school debt, have a mediocre associate job, take on more personal debt, more business debt, and then finally make money…married, kids, house, cars, etc. We then spend and spend to make up for lost time, and assume we make enough that eventually we will save enough. The problem is that we live on false money—inappropriate debt—and we tend to procrastinate true financial responsibility.

If you had to start from scratch building a practice and you could choose either your clinical skills to be in the top 10% of dentists or your communication/leadership skills to be in the top 10% of dentists, which would you choose and why?

Communication skills. Great communication skills can make the difference between failure and extreme success. Also, great communication skills add joy and health to every part of our lives and relationships. Learning better clinical skills is a never-ending practice of ours, and is natural for us to attempt to do. Communication skill improvements are difficult for most of us, yet our skills in that area affect nearly every part of our lives.

Looking back, what advice would you give yourself on the day of your dental school graduation?

I would tell myself to audit much more frequently and hire coaches along the way to help me accomplish very specific goals. I started my first practice right out of school. I would definitely do that all over again.

But I would need to have a strong long-term strategy, medium-term goals, and immediate-term coaches to help propel me on the path. Of course, I can't forget the core issue...I would want to define WHY I do any of this to begin with. Instead of making my work or my profession my WHY, I would tell myself to choose a meaningful WHY outside of work. Make work the means to achieve my real WHY.

When you hear the word success who or what comes to mind?

A person who has found healthy levels of time, money, health, family, community, and spirituality. I equate all of this then to actual long-lasting happiness.

Looking back, can you recognize any pivotal points or revelations on your journey to success? Was there ever a point where you had a clear choice to make and it really determined your path from that point forward?

I remember when I had my first practice seeing 350 new patients per month with 4 dentists, and I wanted to expand. It took me a while to make that decision...but I finally decided yes. Little did I know I would build 10 more practices for myself and see different levels of failure in all of them. It's this process of growth, during this point in my career, where I was able to learn some extremely valuable lessons and put my thinking into an entirely new perspective about the business side of dentistry.

The failures I saw weren't really failures...only through these moments could I finally see the real answers. Without these moments, I would still be far off of the correct path.

If you had to narrow it down to a few key areas, what would you say separates your practice from the hypothetical one down the street doing half the amount of business?

Excellent systemized patient experience, high performance on phones, split-tested marketing, clean financials, patient-friendly payments, high online reviews, smart scheduling, and a focus on quality dentistry, which drives many of our decisions.

In your opinion, what separates the top 10% of dentists from the bottom 90%?

The unique combination of emotional maturity, a strong drive for success, positive attitude, yet a humble and transparent look at their own faults and failures.

What is the best business advice you ever received?

Many times it's just as much work and time to go after 5 zeros as it is to go after 8 zeros. Think bigger and learn from your scaling mistakes. In the end, you only need one success event.

What's something you believe that others may think is crazy?

I believe that we must take out a significant amount of our productive time and replace that with planning and strategy time. Without time for planning and strategic thinking, we end up working really hard doing the wrong thing.

Dave: *I learned this by accident. In 2017, I decided to go from 4-day work weeks in the practice to 3-day work weeks. I wanted more time to work on the business and other projects that I enjoy (like writing this book). My "realistic" goal was to maintain the same production on fewer days. In reality, we grew by 15%. My team and I had more planning, project, and strategy time. Too often, I work harder when the answer is working smarter.*

What does your morning routine look like (let's say, the first hour of the day)?

5:30am – wake up, run a 5K
6:00am – shower, get ready, change a diaper
6:20am – wake up 3 of my 5 kids, get them ready for school.

7:00am – fix 3 kids breakfast

7:15am – drop them off at school

7:30am – arrive at work (first 60min of work has nothing scheduled)

8:30am – start my regularly scheduled meetings

...

3:00pm – end my work day

What book or books have had the most profound impact on your life, business, and otherwise?

Scaling Up: Mastering the Rockefeller Habits 2.0 by Verne Harnish

The 21 Irrefutable Laws of Leadership by John Maxwell

Please explain the most challenging time in your career and how you moved past it and thrived on the other side?

I took on too many dental offices at one time in my call center. We then maxed out our phone technology; our claims clearing house vendor closed their company; and we outgrew our reporting platform...all at once. I underestimated the strain that volume puts on outside vendors and technology, and completely underestimated the lasting affect it would have on my company and people.

If you had to double your prices and couldn't do any paid advertising, what would you focus on to grow your practice?

Phones and case acceptance...without a doubt.

Do you have a favorite quote or mantra you live by?

The only thing that matters is what I choose. I choose to be happy. I choose to do the right thing. I choose to be healthy. I choose to be a good father and husband. I choose to be the person I want to be and have the life I want to have. For some, actually making the choice is hard. Therefore, I focus heavily on what I choose and my own ability to follow it.

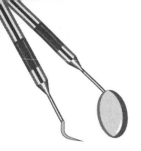

DR. STEFFANY MOHAN

Plaza Dental Group

Dave: *Steffany was one of my first podcast guests. She later invited me out to her practice in Iowa, and that was my introduction to implant dentistry. She's a strong leader, a savvy marketer, a talented educator, and a passionate clinician.*

Background

Dr. Steffany Mohan has practiced dentistry since 1996. She completed her undergraduate work in agricultural biochemistry before earning her Doctorate of Dental Surgery at the University of Iowa.

Since then, Dr. Mohan has built and sold several dental practices and currently owns 3 busy and successful practices in the state of Iowa where she employs 7 associate dentists and 34 team members, including 10 full-time hygienists. She enjoys implementing proven systems in the practices and marketing dentistry.

Dr. Mohan has been chosen for several clinical and practice management educator positions due to her history of serial implementation successes. Dr. Mohan has a true passion for mentoring and guiding colleagues through her own proven clinical management systems.

She works with individual offices as an advisor for their practices and management systems.

Dr. Mohan likes to think of herself as "the dentist next door." She is always curious to learn and master new things and is a proponent of good old-fashioned work ethic. She has lectured internationally as well as extensively in the United States. Dr. Mohan is married to her husband, Mike. They have 4 children, 2 sons and 2 daughters: Luke, Josh, Camaryn, and Halle.

Please explain your style of practice (practice size, location, procedure mix, etc.)

Main practice is a 14-operatory practice with 6 dentists, located in West Des Moines, Iowa. Other locations in Urbandale and Ames, Iowa. The offices provide a comprehensive dentistry approach including complex restorative, implant, Invisalign, Trudenta, and sleep apnea.

Do you have a favorite success quote or mantra?

Ha, it's not necessarily about success, but my favorite is, "The only difference between genius and stupidity is that genius has its limits."

In regards to your dental career, what would you like your legacy to be, or how would you like to be remembered?

I am thrilled that my kids are considering dentistry. I hope that it means that I have come home and made my job and career seem like something that they would like to put on their list of potentials.

What does success mean to you?

Success to me is about doing the right things for the right people for the right reasons. It's about balance and joy and enjoying the people that we care for and about every day.

What is your morning routine (first 1–2 hrs of the day)?

An ideal day includes a workout first thing and then getting kids to school and getting myself out the door.

What is your biggest fear?

Losing a child.

Please explain the most challenging time in your career and how you moved past it and thrived on the other side?

I think it's all been challenging, but I'm never content to coast, so it increases the number and complexity of challenges. I don't dwell in the past too much; today has new challenges and I love to focus on the future and new challenges. That being said, my most challenging times were when my 4 children were young. It was very stressful to have young children and attempt to feel like I was not losing my mind daily.

What is your goal-setting process?

I have a couple of mentors that hold me accountable. I set daily, monthly, and yearly goals with them. Sticking to them is the hard part, but having accountability partners is key.

What is the best investment you have made either inside your career or outside of dentistry?

Investing in the practices has been an excellent decision. We have also invested in medical group buildings, which has been a great ROI.

Looking back, what advice would you give yourself on the day of your dental school graduation?

Get tons of top-quality CE, and find mentors to discuss difficult cases, situations, and patients. Schedule regular time to meet with those mentors. Also, take one day at a time; tomorrow has enough for itself, no need to look too far ahead in most situations.

In your opinion, what separates the top 10% of dentists from the bottom 90%?

Mindset.

What keeps struggling dentists struggling?

Mindset and getting bogged down in minutia.

Justin: I think an entire book could be written on the topic of minutia. We only have a finite amount of focus on a day-to-day basis, and if you aren't focusing on the right things, it can have a crippling effect on your success. Great answer!

What are the top 3 books every dental practice owner should read?

E-Myth by Michael Gerber
Eat That Frog by Brian Tracy
No BS Direct Marketing by Dan Kennedy

If you had to narrow it down to a couple...what traits or skills do you think are most important in running an uncommonly successful practice?

Grit, persistence, humility.

What is a skill or procedure you've added since graduating from dental school that has had a major positive impact on your practice?

Marketing; it's the top thing that, when done well, is priceless.

What is the best business advice you ever received?

Budget for lean times, and always give back more than you receive.

What leadership advice would you give a dentist who has an ineffective culture in their practice?

Be humble and be able to admit when you don't know the answer. Ask for feedback from the team, and give honesty to get back honesty from them.

Dave: It's often very difficult to say "I don't know" as the leader of the practice and the wearer of the white coat. But, the leadership research shows that leaders who show humility and freely admit to their own shortcomings build the strongest cultures.

What advice would you give a dentist that is struggling with case acceptance?

Keep it simple, discuss what a patient really wants and how to get it for them, and be honest about the limitations of dentistry; nothing lasts forever.

What marketing advice would you give a dentist that is starting out in practice ownership?

Read the top 20 marketing books, get a mentor, and track everything.

What do our dental patients most desire?

Trust.

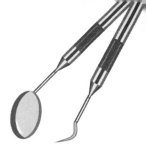

DR. DAVID MALOLEY

Vail Valley Dentist,
The Relentless Dentist Podcast, Author

Background

At his core, David Maloley is a Nebraska farm boy. He attended the University of Nebraska for both undergrad and dental school. His first career pursuit was athletic medicine. He had the incredible experience of working as an athletic trainer under Tom Osborne during Nebraska's football National Championship runs in 1994 and 1995.

Following dental school, He served as an officer in the U.S. Army and was stationed in Germany and Italy. The European experience drove him to find a similar lifestyle near Vail, Colorado. He started Vail Valley Dental Care in 2009 and has been the host of *The Relentless Dentist Podcast* since 2013.

In an effort to give private practice dentists every competitive advantage, he helped launch the Dental Success Network and obtained a High Performance Coach certification. He enjoys skiing, cycling, and exploring the planet with his wife, Karah, and son, Bennett.

Please explain your style of practice (practice size, location, procedure mix, etc.)

I have a small, 4-op general dental practice that I've designed to support our mountain lifestyle and maximize free time. My practice goals are simple: make more and work less each year.

Do you have a favorite success quote or mantra?

"The cave you fear to enter holds the treasure you seek."

—JOSEPH CAMPBELL

In regards to your dental career, what would you like your legacy to be, or how would you like to be remembered?

As the leader of my practice, I want my team to feel like they are better people for having worked there. As a speaker, coach, author, and podcaster, I'd like to be remembered for helping give dentists the courage and confidence to pursue their epic life: a life true to themselves, not the life others expected of them.

What does success mean to you?

Perpetual growth and contribution. Making this year better than last year in every facet of business and life.

What is your morning routine (first 1–2 hrs of the day)?

Wake up around 4:30 or 5. Drink lots of water and take supplements. Meditation for 10–20 minutes. Exercise for 30 minutes. Read, watch, or listen to a thought-provoking book, video, or podcast. Drink a protein shake and a green drink. If I have a strong "mind-body-spirit" morning foundation, I feel like I'm warmed up and ready to take on any challenges that the day may present.

What is your biggest fear?

Deathbed regrets.

Please explain the most challenging time in your career and how you moved past it and thrived on the other side?

I started my practice in 2009. It was a horrible economic time, and I picked a very desirable resort location that had low demand for another dentist. It required all of me to get the practice off the ground. I worked on it day and night. I learned marketing to make the phone ring. I stepped way outside my comfort zone and did live radio and TV spots trying to build a name in the community. I went to Rotary meetings and did elementary school presentations. I was willing to do whatever it took to be successful. Just as I was starting to get some financial footing, my seemingly healthy wife suffered a stroke that almost took her life.

She made a miraculous recovery. But I did not. It was a very financially and emotionally challenging time. I lived in fear of losing my wife and my practice. I was a shell of a man. Because I felt the responsibility to be a good practice owner, husband, and father, I tried to act like everything was okay. Inside I was suffering. I'd get up in the morning barely in enough time to walk in when my first patient arrived. My team rebelled against me during that trying time. Half of them resigned in one week. This was the same team that had given me a card when Karah was in the hospital that said, "We're with you every step of the way." I didn't know who I could trust or turn to.

It was the vision of having an "epic life" in the Rocky Mountains that kept me from giving up completely. It was persistence and clarity of how I wanted my practice to perform and the life I wanted for my family that kept me moving forward. It took years, but I now have the exact lifestyle I blueprinted all those years ago before I moved to Colorado. I go into the office 11–12 days a month. That give me the means and the time to do what I love: skiing 40 days a year, quarterly vacations, and working on fun, impactful business projects like Dental Success Network, speaking at conferences, being a high performance coach for dentists, and writing amazing books like this. :)

What is your goal-setting process?

I have a white board in my home office. It has a grid with 16 sections on it. These sections represent the components that I feel make up an epic life. I use that matrix to make sure I have clarity about where my life is headed. That's my regret-minimization strategy. Using that as a macro-reference, I usually have a number of micro-goals that fit into the grand scheme. They have short-term deadlines ranging from weekly goals to 90-day goals. I like using the Best Self Journal to keep me on track and I have an accountability coach that contacts me weekly to help me determine and follow through on my highest priority tasks.

What is the best investment you have made either inside your career or outside of dentistry?

My dental practice has given me a solid financial return, but the education I've received from starting and operating it has been priceless.

Looking back, what advice would you give yourself on the day of your dental school graduation?

Form strong friendships with like-minded peers that abhor the status quo.

In your opinion, what separates the top 10% of dentists from the bottom 90%?

The top 10% feel fear but choose courage over comfort when making decisions.

What keeps struggling dentists struggling?

They aren't clear on what they want. They avoid taking bold actions that will make them a strong business owner and an assertive leader.

What are the top 3 books every dental practice owner should read?

How to Win Friends and Influence People by Dale Carnegie
The 7 Habits of Highly Effective People by Stephen Covey
The Obstacle is the Way by Ryan Holiday

If you had to narrow it down to a couple...what traits or skills do you think are most important in running an uncommonly successful practice?

Leadership and continuous learning.

What is a skill or procedure you've added since graduating from dental school that has had a major positive impact on your practice?

I used to hate meetings. But now I think the ability to run an effective meeting is critical to unifying a team and getting them to work towards a common cause.

What is the best business advice you ever received?

The masses are asses.

What leadership advice would you give a dentist who has an ineffective culture in their practice?

Start with self-leadership. If you are growing as a person, you'll be much more effective in building a strong culture and helping your individual team members grow. To have more, you need to be more.

What advice would you give a dentist that is struggling with case acceptance?

Case acceptance starts with trust.

What marketing advice would you give a dentist that is starting out in practice ownership?

You're not a dentist. You are a marketer of dental services. Examine every element of your dental practice and ask yourself this question: "Does this add or subtract from the patient experience?" For advertising to work well, you must first have a consistent patient experience that exceeds their expectations.

What do our dental patients most desire?

Compassion and confidence.

CONCLUSION

As a child in the mid-1980s, I attended a tiny, two-room elementary school in rural Nebraska. Despite being a naive, sheltered farm kid, I had no trouble recognizing greatness the first time I saw it. It came in the form of an NBA basketball player. He had personalized shoes and his tongue hung from his mouth as he soared through the air with the ball. He could dominate a slam dunk contest and take over a game in the final minutes despite an entire defense trying to stop him. Of course, I'm talking about #23, Michael Jordan. Over 30 years ago, he sparked an insatiable curiosity in me about greatness. More specifically, the interest was about, "What does it take to rise to the top?"

In that 3-plus decades of study, I've read hundreds of books, watched numerous documentaries, and listened to countless podcasts. I searched for common themes in what made elite athletes, entrepreneurs, leaders, speakers, and performers. In fact, that sense of wonder was one of my motivations to start *The Relentless Dentist Podcast* in 2013.

Fast forward to February 11, 2017. I was on a family vacation (just like Justin was) to get away from the snow for awhile. I was sitting in a bungalow on the shores of the Pacific in Costa Rica. I was reading Tim Ferriss' new book *Tools of the Titans* as I sipped my morning coffee. Yet another exploration of what it takes to get and stay at the top of the game.

Just then my phone buzzed, alerting me to an incoming email. I opened my inbox and saw the subject line: Interview #1: Dr. Dave Maloley The 'Original' RELENTLESS DENTIST. It caught me off guard and so

I quickly opened it. I soon realized it was the interview I had recently done with Dr. Justin Short.

Thanks to the creative inspiration from the Tim Ferriss' book (and the caffeine), I quickly recognized the interview format resembled the interviews I was reading in Tools of the Titans. So I sent an immediate email response to Justin.

The series of emails that would follow initiated a big project that would explore what it takes to reach the top of the dental profession specifically. Now you hold it in your hands, as a reference for how to level up when times are good and how to get unstuck when times are challenging.

In Dr. Lane Ochi's section, he highlighted a quote by Louis Pasteur that said, "Chance favors only the prepared mind." It's an honor to present you this book. It came about by a series of chance events. But it was the primed and prepared minds of Dr. Short and me that quickly recognized that this was a work that was needed by the profession. It came about because we both had started long before dental school, studying success in its many forms. It's also a testament to the magic that can come from like-minded professionals connecting and collaborating.

We intentionally profiled a wide variety of dentists. Some are at the beginnings of their career and some are in the twilight. They have varying practice styles, philosophies, and procedure mixes. There are mega- and multi-practice owners and others with smaller, slower-paced solo practices. Many have done significant things outside of clinical practice. Despite no two of these Titans being alike, I discovered five common lessons that were woven within their stories:

1   **A dental license is only your admission ticket to the profession.** Our colleagues who feel stuck are rarely the same ones who continually invest in themselves by taking advanced clinical continuing education, studying the business of dentistry, or developing as a leader. One of our Titans, Dr. Nate Jeal, once told me,

"I love dentistry because it has no upper limit." I agree. But even though we recognize there's no upper limit, isn't it fun to try to explore it? Titans are continuous learners—they do what others won't, so they've achieved what others can't.

2   **Dentistry can be lonely, but it doesn't have to be.** Finding professional mentors, coaches, peers, and even mentees to support you and your career helps limit the challenges and steepen the learning curve. Titans understand that self-reliance has its limits.

3   **Influence is a learnable skill.** It doesn't matter if you were the bottom of your class or painfully shy (I was both); continually developing your ability to communicate is a key element to growth in this profession. It affects everything from case acceptance to the ability to lead a team. Titans recognize that to make an impact on their families, friends, communities, patients, and profession, they need to promote trust in those relationships.

4   **Hardship is part of the process.** I personally suffered from "why me?" syndrome for the first half of my career. I wondered why the profession had dealt me a bad hand and why so many of my professional heroes seemed to have a path paved with gold. I was just being ignorant. As you've read, sleepless nights, clinical failures, financial setbacks, and personal challenges come with the territory, but Titans turn those obstacles into opportunities.

5   **"Success" is a customizable term.** It's to be defined by the creator of that success. I believe this is critically important to note, because many of us have been caught in the trap of chasing someone else's vision and version of success. Simply pursuing more for more's sake rarely leads to a positive outcome, unless it's connected to a compelling "why". These Titans define success in their own unique way...you should too!

Use those lessons and the innumerable others contained in this book as a guide to future growth, prosperity, and fulfillment. We'll forever be grateful for these Titans of Dentistry for being generous with their time. They were thoughtful and genuine with their observations. Their priceless insights should help us all see our careers with more optimism and possibility.

I feel it is appropriate to conclude this book with homage to one of its major influences:

> *"It is my hope that when you read and reread this book,*
> *you will feel the spirit of these titans with you.*
> *No matter the hardship, challenge, or grand*
> *ambition before you, they are here. You are not*
> *alone, and you are better than you think."*
>
> —TIM FERRISS, *TOOLS OF THE TITANS*

—DR. DAVID MALOLEY, THE RELENTLESS DENTIST

APPENDIX

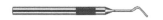

Many books were recommended by Titans. Here is a list of all the recommended books, with the most-recommended appearing first. The number of recommendations appears in parentheses, if more than one dentist recommended a book. Some books at the end were not listed in the "top three books" questions, but were otherwise referenced positively or quoted from.

Books Suggested Inside Titans of Dentistry

Good to Great by Jim Collins (6)

How to Win Friends and Influence People by Dale Carnegie (5)

The E-Myth or *The E-Myth Revisited* by Michael Gerber (4)

Think and Grow Rich by Napoleon Hill (3)

The 7 Habits of Highly Effective People by Stephen Covey (3)

Leaders Eat Last by Simon Sinek (3)

Start With Why by Simon Sinek (3)

Find Your Why by Simon Sinek (2)

The Obstacle Is The Way by Ryan Holiday (2)

Thinking Fast and Slow by Daniel Kahneman (2)

The Tipping Point by Malcolm Gladwell (2)

The Success Principles by Jack Canfield (2)

The Pumpkin Plan by Mike Michalowicz (2)

Rich Dad Poor Dad by Richard Kiyosaki

The 10x Rule by Grant Cardone

Grit by Angela Duckworth

The 4 Disciplines of Execution by Stephen Covey

The Ultimate Sales Machine by Chet Holmes

Relentless by Tim Grover

Small is the New Big by Seth Godin

The Dip by Seth Godin

Stoicism: A Stoic Approach to Modern Life by Tom Miles

The Big Leap by Gay Hendricks

The Checklist Manifesto by Atul Gawande

Eat That Frog by Brian Tracy

The Year of Yes by Shonda Rhimes

The Fred Factor and *The Fred Factor 2.0* by Mark Sanborn

Emotional Intelligence 2.0 by Bradbury and Greaves

The Wow Factor by Tom Peters

Uncommon by Tony Dungy

When Breath Becomes Air by Paul Kalanithi

The Little Book of Common Sense Investing by John Bogle

The Bible by God and Various Authors

Functional Occlusion by Peter Dawson

Who Moved My Cheese by Ken Blanchard

Sell or Be Sold by Grant Cardone

One Minute Manager by Blanchard and Johnson

Don't Wait for the Tooth Fairy: How to Communicate by Ashley Latter

Drive by Daniel Pink

Flip Your Focus by Bob Spiel

Team of Teams by Gen. McChrystal

Scaling Up: Mastering the Rockefeller Habits 2.0 by Verne Harnish

The 21 Irrefutable Laws of Leadership by John Maxwell

The Millionaire Next Door by Thomas Stanley

The Answer by John Assaraf

Integrity Selling for the 21st Century by Ron Willingham

Change your Questions, Change Your Life by Marilee Adams

The Art of Possibility by Rosamund Zander

The Energy of Money by Maria Nemeth

The Philosophy of the Practice of Dentistry by Pankey and Davis

Extreme Ownership by Jocko Willink and Leif Babin

Built to Sell by John Warrillow

The Magic of Thinking Big by David Schwartz

The New Psychology of Achievement by Brian Tracy

The Power of the Subconscious Mind by Joseph Murphy

Megatrends by John Naisbitt

The Great Game of Business by Jack Stack

No B.S. Direct Marketing by Dan Kennedy

Making it Easy for Patients to say "Yes" by Paul Homoly

Expert Secrets by Russel Brunson

Bonded Porcelain Restorations by Pascal Magne

The Only Guide to a Winning Investment Strategy You'll Ever Need by Larry Swedroe

Making Money Is Killing Your Business by Chuck Blakeman

The Subtle Art of Not Giving a F*ck by Mark Manson

Mastery by Robert Greene

Successful Preventive Dental Practices by Bob Barkley

Where Good Ideas Come From by Steven Johnson

The seminar manual from Breakaway

Implant Excellence by Arun Garg

Everything is Marketing by Fred Joyal

The 4-Hour Workweek by Tim Ferriss

Tools of the Titans by Tim Ferriss

The Artist's Way by Julia Cameron

Break From the Pack by Oren Harari

ACKNOWLEDGEMENTS

We want to extend a very heartfelt Thank You to all the Titans that contributed your time and wisdom to share with others. Without you, this book wouldn't have been possible. We are very grateful.

—DRS. SHORT & MALOLEY

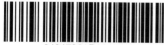

34847321R00176

Made in the USA
Columbia, SC
17 November 2018